McMinn's Color Atlas of
Lower Limb
Anatomy

McMinn's Color Atlas of
Lower Limb
Anatomy
Fifth Edition

Bari M. Logan MA FMA Hon MBIE MAMAA

Formerly University Prosector, Department of Anatomy, University of Cambridge, UK; Prosector, Department of Anatomy,
The Royal College of Surgeons of England, London, UK and Anatomical Preparator, Department of Human Morphology,
University of Nottingham Medical School, UK

David J. Bowden MA Vet MB MB BChir FRCR

Consultant Radiologist, Cambridge University Hospitals, Cambridge, UK

Original Photography by Ralph T. Hutchings

Photographer for Visuals Unlimited.com
Formerly Chief Medical Laboratory Scientific Officer, The Royal College of Surgeons of England, London, UK

Regional Anaesthesia by:

Anand M. Sardesai MBBS MD DA FRCA
    Consultant Anaesthetist
Sachin Daivajna MBBS MS MRCS
    Specialist Registrar
A. H. N. Robinson BSc FRCS (Orth)
    Consultant Orthopaedic Surgeon, Cambridge University Hospitals, Cambridge, UK

ELSEVIER

ELSEVIER

Notices

Knowledge and best practice in this field are constantly changing. As new research and experience broaden our understanding, changes in research methods, professional practices, or medical treatment may become necessary.

Practitioners and researchers must always rely on their own experience and knowledge in evaluating and using any information, methods, compounds, or experiments described herein. In using such information or methods they should be mindful of their own safety and the safety of others, including parties for whom they have a professional responsibility.

With respect to any drug or pharmaceutical products identified, readers are advised to check the most current information provided (i) on procedures featured or (ii) by the manufacturer of each product to be administered, to verify the recommended dose or formula, the method and duration of administration, and contraindications. It is the responsibility of practitioners, relying on their own experience and knowledge of their patients, to make diagnoses, to determine dosages and the best treatment for each individual patient, and to take all appropriate safety precautions.

To the fullest extent of the law, neither the Publisher nor the authors, contributors, or editors, assume any liability for any injury and/or damage to persons or property as a matter of products liability, negligence or otherwise, or from any use or operation of any methods, products, instructions, or ideas contained in the material herein.

ISBN: 978-0-7020-7218-5

Printed in Great Britain

Last digit is the print number: 9 8 7 6 5 4 3

ELSEVIER | your source for books, journals and multimedia in the health sciences

www.elsevierhealth.com

Working together to grow libraries in developing countries

www.elsevier.com • www.bookaid.org

The publisher's policy is to use paper manufactured from sustainable forests

Content Strategist: Jeremy Bowes
Content Development Specialist: Carole McMurray
Project Manager: Andrew Riley
Design: Maggie Reid
Illustration Manager: Amy Faith Heyden
Marketing Manager: Deborah Watkins

Contents

Dedications

To Arlette Herzig and Robert Logan
- Bari Logan

Anna, Jack, George and my parents
- David Bowden

Anne, Sam and Isabel
- Ralph Hutchings

And

To the Memory of an Esteemed Colleague

Professor R. M. H. (Bob) McMinn

Preface

This fifth edition of *McMinn's Colour Atlas of Foot and Ankle Anatomy*, heralds 35 years of publication and brings some significant changes and most immediate to note is the new title, **McMinn's Color Atlas of Lower Limb Anatomy**, which we feel reflects more truly the overall direction and content of the book.

Originally intended as an illustrated reference book for chiropodists and podiatrists in training, over the ensuing years it has become equally popular with radiologists, physiotherapists, sports injury consultants, vascular and orthopaedic surgeons. The book has therefore become an accepted standard text on the subject and continues to fill an important niche on medical library bookshelves worldwide, producing eight language editions: English, Chinese, Japanese, French, German, Dutch, Russian and Spanish.

For this fifth edition, a third co-author David Bowden joins the team and adds his specialist clinical knowledge and expertise in the field of radiology by adding a new 30 page chapter dedicated to **Imaging of the Lower Limb**, using state-of-the-art technology. Thus providing the opportunity to visualise key anatomical structures as they appear in the living subject in comparison to the illustrations of bones and detailed anatomical preparations provided elsewhere in the book.

Bari Logan adds a scattering of nine new pages of annotated illustrations of anatomical preparations, with accompanying notes.

We hope that these new additions and overall review of the text will be appreciated and that the book will continue in its popularity as an important contribution to medical education at both pre-clinical and postgraduate level.

Bari M Logan
Siegershausen, Switzerland
David J Bowden
Cambridge, UK
March 2017

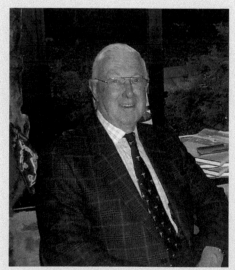

Ardfern – 5 April 2008

Professor R. M. H. McMinn, MD (Glas), PhD (Sheff), FRCS (Eng)
[b. Sept 23, 1923 – d. July 11, 2012, aged 88]

Robert 'Bob' McMinn was a medical graduate of the University of Glasgow. After leaving hospital posts and service with the Royal Air Force in Iraq and Africa, he began his anatomical career as a Demonstrator in Anatomy in Glasgow in 1950. He became a lecturer in the University of Sheffield and was later Reader and then Titular Professor at King's College, London. In 1970 he was appointed to the Chair of Anatomy at the Royal College of Surgeons of England. Among his publications, 'A Colour Atlas of Human Anatomy', with photographer R. T. Hutchings, was first published in 1977 and became a worldwide best seller, with translations into over 25 languages; more than 4 million copies were sold.

For this and other later atlases his co-authors added the name 'McMinn' to the titles in recognition of his contribution to anatomical teaching. He was editor of the eighth and ninth editions of 'Last's Anatomy Regional and Applied', which remains a standard work for surgical trainees. He was program secretary and later treasurer of the Anatomical Society of Great Britain and Ireland, and was a founder member and first secretary of the British Association of Clinical Anatomists. At the International Anatomical Congress held in Cambridge in 2000, he received a Special Presentation Award from the Anatomical Society for his teaching and research activities. His research interests were in wound healing and tissue repair and on the association between skin disease and the alimentary tract.

He retired in 1983 and moved with his wife back to their Scottish homeland settling on the west coast in Ardfern, Lochgilphead.

McMinn's Legacy of Illustrated Anatomy Books

Bari Logan entered the academic post of Prosector to the department of Anatomy, The Royal College of Surgeons, of England, London, in January 1977. At that time, 'Bob' McMinn held the Chair as Sir William Collins Professor of Human and Comparative Anatomy and Ralph Hutchings was the Chief Medical Scientific Officer and departmental photographer.

In April of the same year, an evening reception was held at the College for a group of distinguished medical fraternity by Wolfe Medical Publications to launch a new book entitled *A Colour Atlas of Human Anatomy* by the authors McMinn & Hutchings who had spent the previous 2 years working on the project.

1977 - ISBN 0-7234-0709-6
2ⁿᵈ Ed—1988
3ʳᵈ Ed—1993
4ᵗʰ Ed—1998
5ᵗʰ Ed—2003
6ᵗʰ Ed—2008
7ᵗʰ Ed—2013

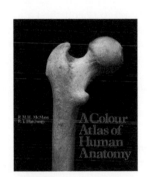

First Edition dust cover wrap

Instantly considered by many to be a visually stunning production, it was without doubt a pioneering book in the field of human anatomy, having many novel concepts in both composition and design that would later be adopted by other authors and become standard format in many new illustrated texts on the subject.

The book, 352 pages, was unusually large in size and contained over 700 high quality colour photographs of almost natural size, bones, detailed dissections (prosections), and exquisite anatomical preparations depicting the entire human body taken of specimens hitherto unseen beyond the closely guarded confines of the dissecting room and anatomical museum. Essentially designed as a general reference work for the medical profession, the book rapidly became a best-seller, quickly producing 25 foreign language editions and attaining over 4 million copies in sales worldwide, it won numerous awards and gained much international academic acclaim.

The book remains in print today, 40 years on and in its seventh edition (2013), but since the fourth edition, under entirely new

authorship, direction and content, although the name 'McMinn' remains in the title for posterity.

Following on from the enormous success of *A Colour Atlas*, the publisher Peter Wolfe approached 'Bob' McMinn and Ralph Hutchings in early 1979 with the idea of producing a new illustrated text to suit the specific educational needs of dental students, for whom the Royal College of Surgeons ran popular postgraduate courses.

Wolfe's proposal was timely because, within the College, the renovation and reorganization of the Wellcome Museum of Anatomy and Physiology, founded by the famous Australian anatomist R. (Ray) J. Last in (1947), was well underway; a particular pressing need, identified by Bari Logan, was to prepare for display a range of detailed head and neck prosections and preparations, for which the collection was lacking.

Thus, the co-authorship trio of McMinn, Hutchings and Logan was formed and within a two-year period produced their first book together in 1981.

1981: ISBN 0-7234-0755-X
A Colour Atlas of Head and Neck Anatomy
Wolfe Medical Publications: McMinn/Hutchings/Logan
Designed for dental students
English, French, German, Italian, Japanese, Korean, Portuguese, Spanish
2ⁿᵈ Ed—1994
3ʳᵈ Ed—2004
4ᵗʰ Ed—2009
5ᵗʰ Ed—2017

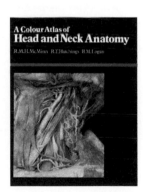

Over the next 17 years, there followed a fairly rapid succession of books, despite the retirement of Ralph Hutchings in 1981, 'Bob' McMinn in 1983, academic career move of Bari Logan to Cambridge in 1987 and further complications along the way of various changes to publishers through company takeovers, each having additional authorship commitments on other new books.

Key to this speedy turnover was the ability to combine individual talent in a very harmonious way, work to a logical regime and keep within a strict timeframe whilst always maintaining an essential keen eye for detail.

1982: ISBN 0-7234-0782-7
A Colour Atlas of Foot and Ankle Anatomy
Wolfe Medical Publications: McMinn/Hutchings/Logan
Designed for Podiatrists and Chiropodists
English, Chinese, Dutch, French, German, Japanese, Russian, Spanish
2nd Ed—1995
3rd Ed—2004
4th Ed—2012
5th Ed—2017 **Lower Limb Anatomy**

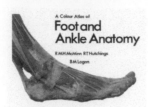

1984: ISBN 0-7234-0831-9
A Colour Atlas of Applied Anatomy
Wolfe Medical Publications: McMinn/Hutchings/Logan
Designed for clinicians (The anatomy of approaches for surgical and clinical procedures.)
English, Japanese
Out of Print

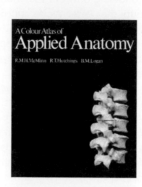

1986: ISBN 0-7234-0911-0
Picture Tests in Human Anatomy
Wolfe Medical Publications: McMinn/Hutchings/Logan
Designed for medical students taking practical exams
English, French, German, Japanese, Portuguese, Serbo-Croatian, Spanish
Out of Print

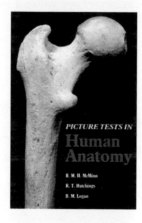

1986: ISBN 0-7234-0958-7
The Human Skeleton: a Photographic Manual in Colour
Wolfe Medical Publications: McMinn/Hutchings/Logan
Designed for medical students (fold down, full size skeleton pictures and individual bones)
English, Danish, French, German, Greek, Japanese, Portuguese, Spanish
2nd Edition—2007

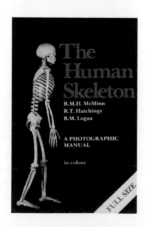

1995: ISBN 0-7234-0967-6
McMinn's Functional and Clinical Anatomy
Mosby: McMinn/Gaddum-Rosse/Hutchings/Logan
Designed for medical students
English, Italian, Greek
Out of Print

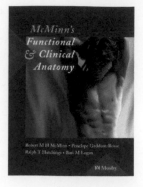

Functional and Clinical, included a fourth co-author, Penelope Gaddum-Rosse, a distinguished physiologist, and work began on the project in 1987 as a text originally intended for the nursing profession and appropriately entitled, *Anatomy and Physiology for Nurses,* with the publishers Wolfe.

However, following a takeover of Wolfe Medical Publications by Mosby Year Book Europe, who already had an extensive nursing book list which included both, physiology and anatomy titles, the manuscript was shelved for a number of years until a decision on its fate was finally reached in 1993 with the proposal for 'Bob' McMinn to re-edit the entire text and tailor it more to the needs of pre-clinical and postgraduate medical students. 'Bob' completed the task in just under one year and, interestingly, it is considered to be the best written of all the McMinn books.

Their final book together was published in 1998.

1998: ISBN 1-874545-52-9
The Concise Handbook of Human Anatomy
Manson Publishing: McMinn/Hutchings/Logan
Designed for sixth form students entering a medical career
English, German, Portuguese
2nd Ed—2017
McMinn's Concise Human Anatomy
CRC Press (Taylor & Francis)
Heylings/Carmichael/Leinster/Saada

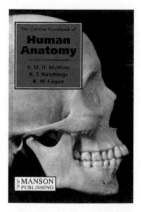

'Bob' was the inspirational driving force behind each book and, from start of the project, would clearly outline overall content and specific illustrative requirements for each chapter producing rough sketches or photocopies with accompanying detailed lists of all the most important anatomical structures needed to be clearly seen in the resulting pictures.

Bari would interpret this information, produce his own notes and drawings and carry out the various detailed prosections or anatomical preparations working to the specific camera lens angle and overall framed view required.

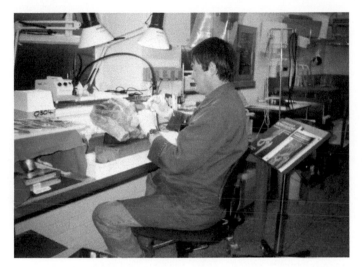

Bari M. Logan, Prosector

Sporadic photographic sessions were held, often late evenings and weekends, under the 'eagle eye' of 'Bob' who would advise on the camera angle and ensure that all the structures essential to identify were displayed in their correct anatomical positions.

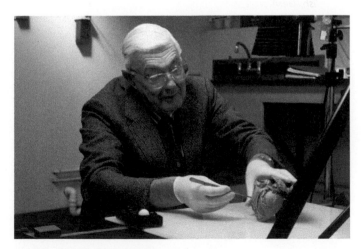

Professor R. ('Bob') H. McMinn, Anatomist

Ralph spent infinite time setting-up lighting, establishing correct camera exposure settings and, by using full format colour film, produced images of exceptional quality and depth in detail.

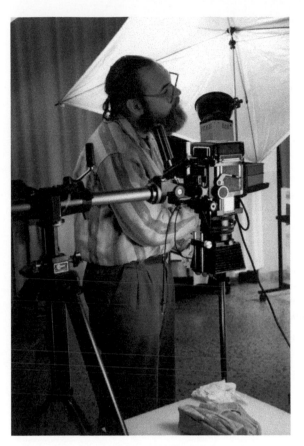

Ralph T. Hutchings, Photographer

Since the first publication, over the ensuing 36 years to date (2017), the seven books produced by the trio, have thus far, created 17 English editions and 13 foreign language editions: Chinese, Danish, Dutch, French, German, Greek, Italian, Japanese, Korean, Portuguese, Russian, Serbo-Croation and Spanish, with total sales exceeding well over 1 million copies worldwide.

Four of the books remain popular and still in print: *Head & Neck, 5th edition*; *Foot & Ankle, 5th edition,* now more appropriately retitled *Lower Limb Anatomy*; *Human Skeleton, 2nd edition*; and the *Concise Handbook – 2nd edition*, which now has a new publisher and authorship, and to conform with the other surviving publications 'McMinns' prefixed in the title.

Overall, a remarkable literary achievement in such a specialized field and only made possible by the unique visionary authorship and guidance of 'Bob' McMinn, whose legacy of Illustrated books on the subject of human anatomy has not only made a significant contribution to medical education in general, but also to the grateful appreciation and applause of thousands of aspiring students throughout the world.

Bari Logan and Ralph Hutchings
June 2016

Acknowledgements

The authors are indebted to the following:

- Prof Adrian Dixon, Prof Harold Ellis and Dr Robert Whitaker for help and expert advice on lower limb lymphatics.
- Dr Ian G. Parkin, Clinical Anatomist, University of Cambridge UK, for expert anatomical knowledge.
- Anand Sardesai, Sachin Daivajna and A. Robinson of Addenbrooke's Hospital Cambridge, for jointly providing the excellent chapter on 'Regional Anaesthesia for Ankle and Foot'.
- Mel Lazenby, Lucie Whitehead and the late Martin Watson (2008), Department of Anatomy, University of Cambridge UK, for the preservation of anatomical material.
- Adrian Newman, Ian Bolton and John Bashford, Anatomy Visual Media Group (AVMG), Department of Physiology, Developmental Neuroscience, University of Cambridge UK, for new edition photographs and digital expertise.

Radiographs

- Dr Oscar Craig p.21B.
- Dr Kate Stevens p.31C.

Illustrations on pages 24–25 and 90–91 are reproduced with permission from *Logan's Illustrated Human Anatomy—A Pictorial Introduction to Basic Form and Structure,* B.M.Logan (CRC Press 2016); and on pages 34-37 from *Human Sectional Anatomy–Atlas of Body Sections, CT and MRI Images, 4th Edition,* H.Ellis, B.M.Logan, A.K.Dixon and D.J.Bowden (CRC Press 2015).

Gluteal intramuscular injection on page 25 is reproduced with permission from *McMinn's Functional and Clinical Anatomy,* R.M.H.McMinn, P.Gaddum-Rosse, R.T.Hutchings and B.M.Logan (Mosby 1995).

Dissection/anatomical preparation credits
The following individuals are credited for their skilled in preparing the following anatomical material illustrated in this book:
  Mrs Carmen Bester: page 90A.
  Bari M Logan: pages 2B, 4B, 6B, 8B, 10, 12, 14A, 16A, 17B, 20A, 24A, 25B, 26A, 27C, 28A, 29B, 31D, 34, 35A, 36B, 37C, 38A, 40ABC, 41DEF, 74A, 75BC, 76A, 77B, 78, 80A, 81B, 82A, 83B, 84, 86AB, 88, 92A, 93B, 94A, 95B, 96AB, 97C, 98A, 99B, 100A, 101B, 102A, 103B, 104ABC, 106AB, 108ΛB, 110AB, 111AB, and 112ABCDE.
  Ms Lynette Nearn: pages 91B, 166.
  Dr David H Tompsett: pages 30B, 33BC and 39D.

Terminology

The Greek adjective 'peroneal' is now replaced by the Latin 'fibular' for various muscles, vessels, nerves, and structures; For example: **Fibularis tertius** instead of Peroneus tertius; **Fibular artery** instead of Peroneal artery; **Common fibular nerve** instead of Common peroneal nerve; **Inferior fibular retinaculum** instead of Inferior peroneal retinaculum.

Again, for this new edition, to ease in the new terminology for those used to working from older texts, the term *peroneal* is included italicized in brackets, e.g., **Deep fibular** (peroneal) **nerve**.

Also note, Flexor accessorius is now known as **quadratus plantae.**

This terminology conforms to the International Anatomical Terminology—Terminologia Anatomica—created in 1988 by the Federative Committee on Anatomical Terminology (FCAT) and approved by the 56 Member Associations of the International Federation of Associations of Anatomists (IFAA). Stuttgart: Thieme ISBN 3-13-115251-6.

Preservation of Cadavers

Long-term preservation of the cadavers, utilized for the majority of anatomical dissections (prosections) illustrated in this book, was by standard embalming technique, using an electric motor pump set at a constant pressure rate of 15 p.s.i. Perfusion was achieved through the arterial system via femoral artery cannulation of one leg and return drainage of the accompanying vein.

On acceptance of 20 litres of preservative fluid by pump, local injection of those areas not visibly affected was carried out by automatic syringe.

On average, 30 litres of preservative fluid was used to preserve each cadaver.

Immediately following embalming, cadavers were encapsulated in thick-gauge, clear polythene bags and cold stored at a temperature of 10.6° C at 40 percent humidity for a minimum period of 16 weeks before dissection. This period of storage allowed preservative fluid to thoroughly saturate the body tissues, resulting in a highly satisfactory state of preservation.

The chemical formula for the preservative fluid (Logan *et al.*, 1989) is:

Methylated spirit 64 over proof	12.5 litres
Phenol liquefied 80%	2.5 litres
Formaldehyde solution 38%	1.5 litres
Glycerine BP	3.5 litres
	Total = 20 litres

The resultant working strength of each constituent is:

Methylated spirit	55%
Glycerine	12%
Phenol	10%
Formaldehyde solution	3%

The advantages of using this particular preservative fluid are:

(1) A state of soft preservation is achieved, benefiting dissection techniques.
(2) The low formaldehyde solution content obviates excessive noxious fumes.
(3) A degree of natural tissue colour is maintained, benefiting photography.
(4) Mould growth does not occur on either whole cadavers thus preserved or their subsequent dissected (prosected) and stored parts.

SAFETY FOOTNOTE

Since the preparation of the anatomical material used in this book, there have been substantial major changes to health and safety regulations concerning the use of certain chemical constituents in preservative (embalming) fluids. It is essential, therefore, to seek official local health and safety advice and guidance if intending to adopt the above preservative fluid.

Orientation Guides

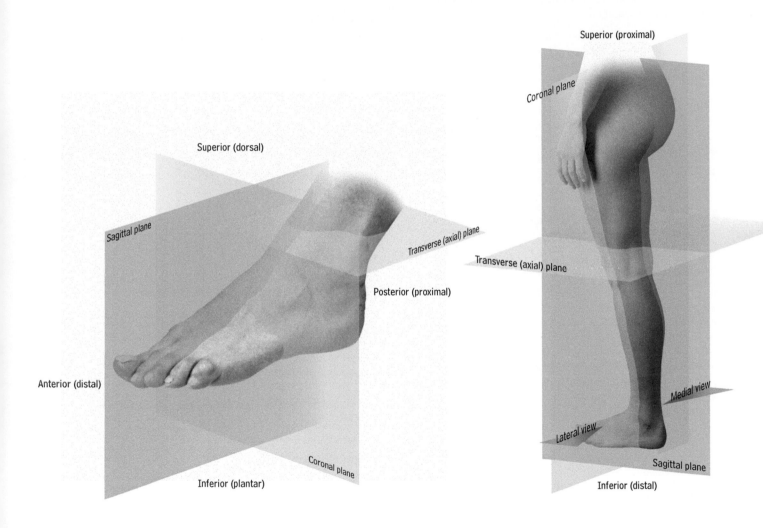

Superior (dorsal)

Sagittal plane

Transverse (axial) plane

Posterior (proximal)

Anterior (distal)

Coronal plane

Inferior (plantar)

Superior (proximal)

Coronal plane

Transverse (axial) plane

Medial view

Lateral view

Sagittal plane

Inferior (distal)

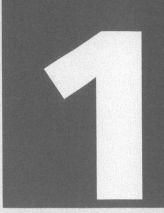

Lower limb, pelvis and hip

Lower limb survey

Bones, muscles and surface landmarks of the left lower limb, from the front

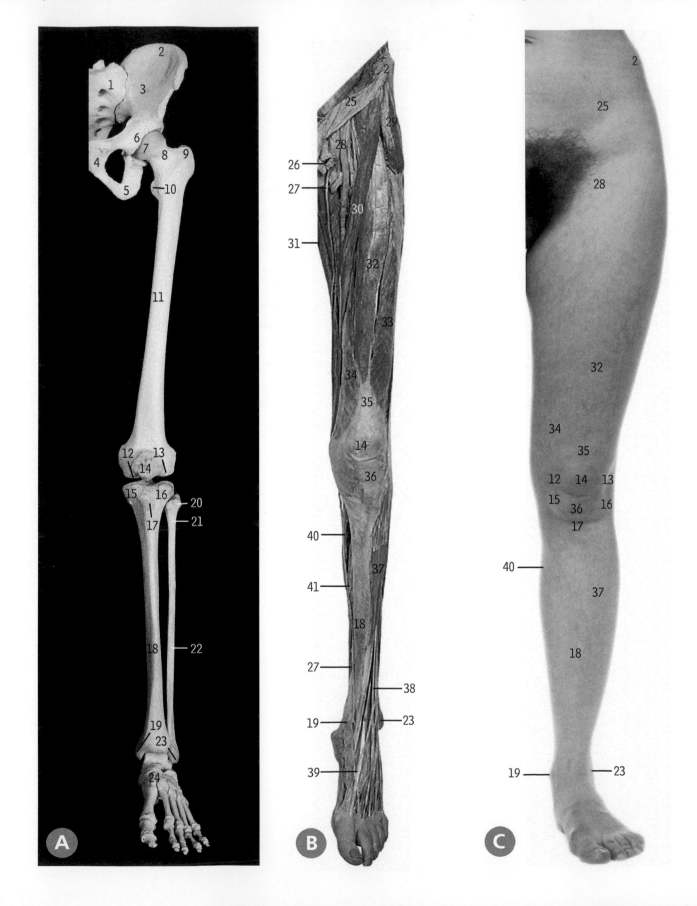

1 Sacrum
2 Iliac crest
3 Ilium ⎫
4 Pubis ⎬ of hip bone
5 Ischium ⎭
6 Rim of acetabulum
7 Head ⎫
8 Neck ⎪
9 Greater trochanter ⎪
10 Lesser trochanter ⎬ of femur
11 Body (shaft) ⎪
12 Medial condyle ⎪
13 Lateral condyle ⎭
14 Patella
15 Medial condyle ⎫
16 Lateral condyle ⎪
17 Tuberosity ⎬ of tibia
18 Body (shaft) ⎪
19 Medial malleolus ⎭
20 Head ⎫
21 Neck ⎬ of fibula
22 Body (shaft) ⎪
23 Lateral malleolus ⎭
24 Foot
25 Inguinal ligament
26 Inguinal lymph nodes
27 Great saphenous vein
28 Femoral triangle, vessels and nerve
29 Tensor fasciae latae
30 Sartorius
31 Gracilis
32 Rectus femoris
33 Vastus lateralis
34 Vastus medialis
35 Quadriceps tendon
36 Patellar ligament
37 Tibialis anterior
38 Extensor digitorum longus
39 Extensor hallucis longus
40 Gastrocnemius
41 Soleus

A Bones of the left lower limb, from the front

B Muscles of the left lower limb, from the front

C Surface landmarks of the left lower limb, from the front

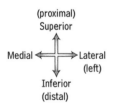

(proximal)
Superior

Medial ⟵⟶ Lateral
(left)

Inferior
(distal)

- The main parts or regions of the lower limb are the gluteal region (consisting of the hip at the side and the buttock at the back), the thigh, the knee, the leg, the ankle and the foot. The term *leg* properly refers to the part between the knee and the foot, although it is commonly used for the whole lower limb.
- The hip bone consists of three bones fused together—the ilium (**3**), ischium (**5**) and pubis (**4**)—and forms a pelvic girdle. The two hip bones or girdles unite with each other in front at the pubic symphysis (p. 18, **B33**), and at the back they join the sacrum at the sacro-iliac joints (p. 18, **A7** and p. 19, **C6**), so forming the bony pelvis.
- The femur (**11**) is the bone of the thigh; the tibia (**18**) and fibula (**22**) are the bones of the leg.
- The acetabulum (**6**) of the hip bone and the head of the femur (**7**) form the hip joint (p. 18, **A12** and **14**, **B18** and **20**, **C18** and **20**).
- The condyles of the femur (**12** and **13**) and tibia (**15** and **16**) together with the patella (**14**) form the knee joint.
- The head of the fibula (**20**) forms a small joint with the tibia, the superior tibiofibular joint. The inferior tibiofibular joint, properly called the tibiofibular syndesmosis (a type of fibrous joint), is a fibrous union between the tibia and fibula just above the ankle joint.
- The ankle is the lower part of the leg in the region of the ankle joint (pp. 60, 62, 64 and 66).
- The lower ends of the tibia (**18**) and fibula (**22**) articulate with the talus of the foot to form the ankle joint (pp. 60 and 62).
- The body of a long bone is commonly called the shaft.
- The adjective 'peroneal' (Greek, see p. 49) is now replaced by the Latin 'fibular' for various vessels and nerves, e.g., common fibular nerve instead of common peroneal nerve. See notes on New Terminology on p. xiii.

- For details of limb muscles, nerves and arteries, see the Appendix:

Muscles—pp. 116–121, including **Figs 2–7**.

Nerves—pp. 122–123, including **Figs 8** and **9**.

Arteries—pp. 136 and 137, including **Figs 27** and **28**.

Lower limb survey

Bones, muscles and surface landmarks of the left lower limb, from behind

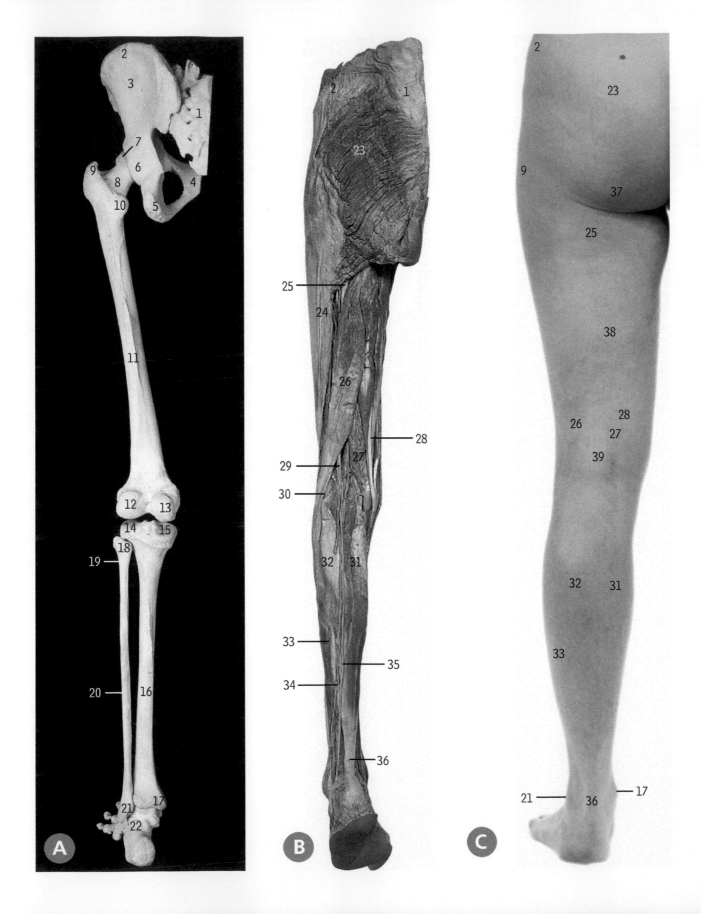

1 Sacrum
2 Iliac crest
3 Ilium
4 Pubis
5 Ischium
6 Rim of acetabulum
7 Head ⎫
8 Neck
9 Greater trochanter
10 Lesser trochanter ⎬ of femur
11 Body
12 Lateral condyle
13 Medial condyle ⎭
14 Lateral condyle ⎫
15 Medial condyle ⎬ of tibia
16 Body
17 Medial malleolus ⎭
18 Head ⎫
19 Neck ⎬ of fibula
20 Body
21 Lateral malleolus ⎭
22 Foot
23 Gluteus maximus
24 Iliotibial tract
25 Sciatic nerve
26 Biceps femoris
27 Semimembranosus
28 Semitendinosus
29 Tibial nerve
30 Common fibular (*peroneal*) nerve
31 Medial head ⎫ of gastrocnemius
32 Lateral head ⎭
33 Soleus
34 Sural nerve
35 Small saphenous vein
36 Tendo calcaneus
37 Fold of buttock (gluteal fold)
38 Hamstring muscles
39 Popliteal fossa

- The curved fold of the buttock (**37**) does not correspond to the straight (but oblique) lower border of gluteus maximus (**23**).
- The tendons of gastrocnemius (**31** and **32**) and soleus (**33**) join to form the tendo calcaneus (**36**), known commonly as the Achilles' tendon.
- The muscles on the back of the thigh with prominent tendons—semimembranosus (**27**), semitendinosus (**28**) and biceps femoris (long head, **26**)—are known commonly as the hamstrings (see the note on p. 29).

(A) **Bones of the left lower limb, from behind**

(B) **Muscles of the left lower limb, from behind**

(C) **Surface landmarks of the left lower limb, from behind**

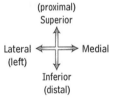

(proximal)
Superior

Lateral ⟵⟶ Medial
(left)

Inferior
(distal)

Lower limb survey

Bones, muscles and surface landmarks of the left lower limb, from the medial side

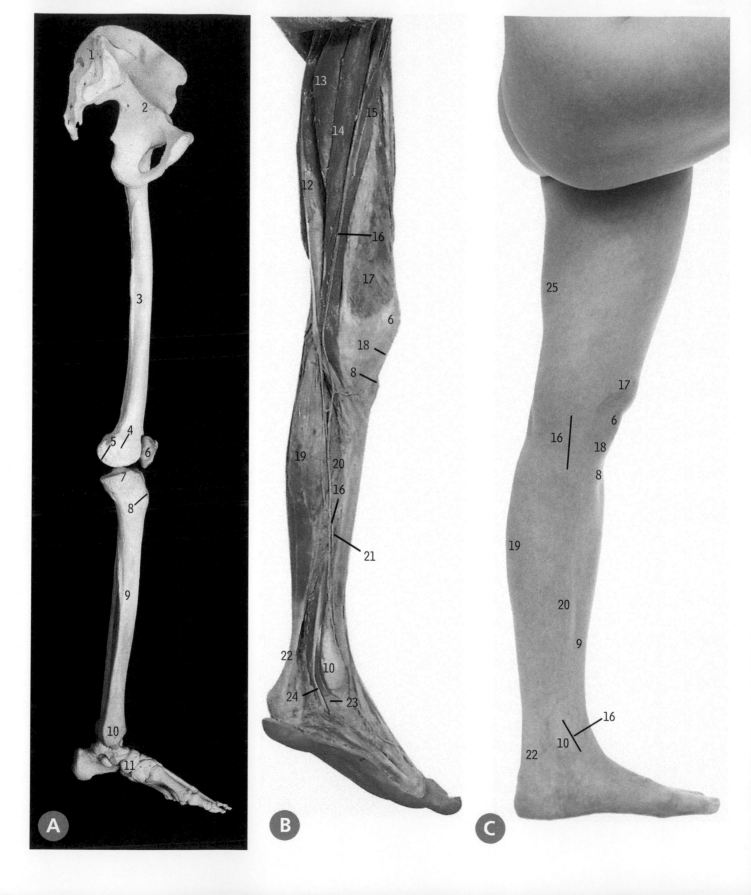

1 Sacrum
2 Hip bone
3 Body ⎫
4 Medial epicondyle ⎬ of femur
5 Medial condyle ⎭
6 Patella
7 Medial condyle ⎫
8 Tuberosity ⎬ of tibia
9 Body ⎪
10 Medial malleolus ⎭
11 Foot
12 Semitendinosus
13 Semimembranosus
14 Gracilis
15 Sartorius
16 Great saphenous vein
17 Vastus medialis
18 Patellar ligament
19 Gastrocnemius
20 Soleus
21 Saphenous nerve
22 Tendo calcaneus
23 Tibialis posterior
24 Flexor digitorum longus
25 Hamstrings

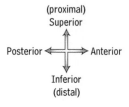

(proximal)
Superior

Posterior ←——→ Anterior

Inferior
(distal)

- At the ankle the great saphenous vein (16), the longest vein in the body, passes upwards in front of the medial malleolus (10). At the knee it lies a hand's breadth behind the medial border of the patella (6). It ends by draining into the femoral vein (p. 24, 12 and 18).

Ⓐ Bones of the left lower limb, from the medial side

Ⓑ Muscles of the left lower limb, from the medial side

Ⓒ Surface landmarks of the left lower limb, from the medial side

Lower limb survey

Bones, muscles and surface landmarks of the left lower limb, from the lateral side

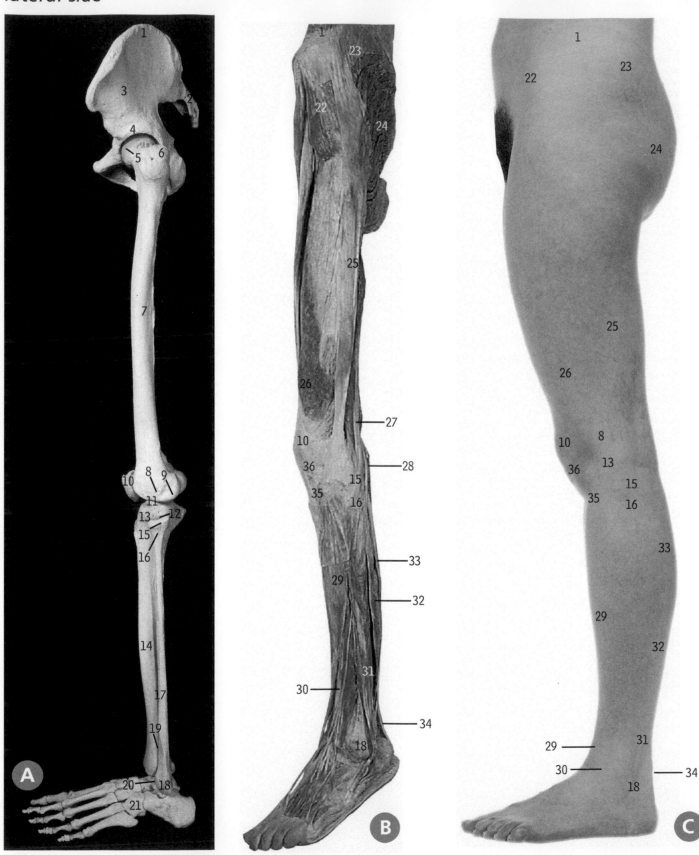

1 Iliac crest
2 Sacrum
3 Hip bone
4 Hip joint
5 Head
6 Greater trochanter
7 Body ⎫ of femur
8 Lateral epicondyle
9 Lateral condyle ⎭
10 Patella
11 Knee joint
12 Superior tibiofibular joint
13 Lateral condyle ⎫ of tibia
14 Body
15 Head ⎫
16 Neck
17 Body ⎬ of fibula
18 Lateral malleolus ⎭
19 Inferior tibiofibular joint
20 Ankle joint
21 Foot
22 Tensor fasciae latae
23 Gluteus medius
24 Gluteus maximus
25 Iliotibial tract
26 Vastus lateralis
27 Biceps femoris
28 Common fibular (*peroneal*) nerve
29 Tibialis anterior
30 Extensor digitorum longus
31 Fibularis (*peroneus*) longus
32 Soleus
33 Gastrocnemius
34 Tendo calcaneus
35 Tibial tuberosity
36 Patellar ligament

- The common fibular (*peroneal*) nerve (**28**), the only *palpable* major nerve of the lower limb, can be felt as it passes downward and forward across the neck of the fibula (**16**).

A Bones of the left lower limb, from the lateral side

B Muscles of the left lower limb, from the lateral side

C Surface landmarks of the left lower limb, from the lateral side

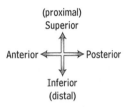

(proximal)
Superior

Anterior ←—→ Posterior

Inferior
(distal)

Male pelvic viscera and vessels

Seen on the right side in a sagittal section, after removal of most of the peritoneum (serous membrane)

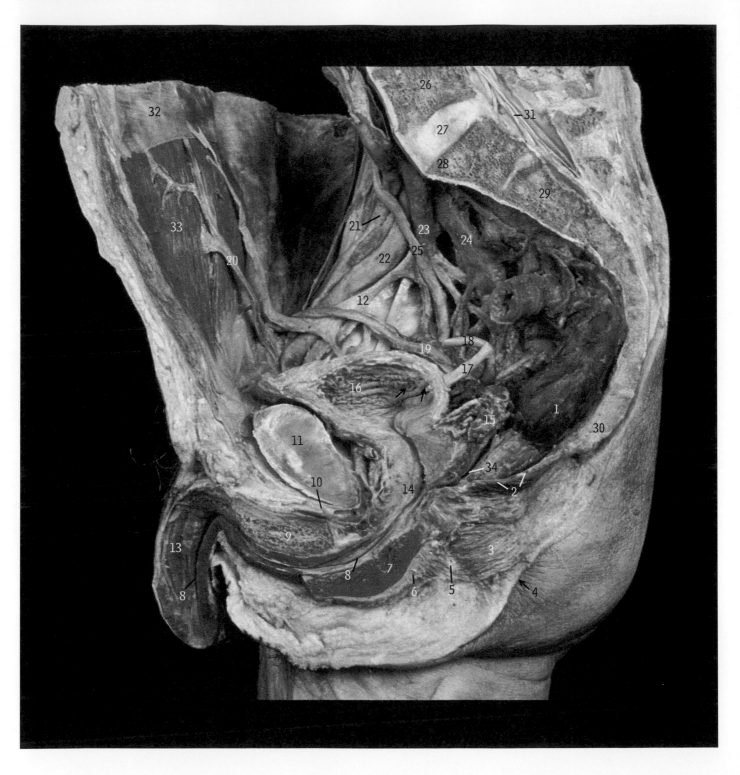

The section is mostly in the midline; small bowel, large bowel and peritoneum (serous membrane) have been removed but the whole of the anal canal and the lower part of the left levator ani muscle have been preserved to show the external anal sphincter (as in the female section, p. 12).

1 Rectum
2 Cut edge of levator ani
3 External anal sphincter covering anal canal
4 Anus, above arrowhead
5 Perineal body
6 Bulbospongiosus overlying corpus spongiosum
7 Corpus spongiosum, the part of the penis containing the urethra
8 Spongy part of urethra, within the corpus spongiosum
9 Corpus cavernosum of penis
10 Deep dorsal vein of penis, draining back to the vesicoprostatic venous plexus, the sponge-like tissue sectioned here in front of the prostate
11 Pubic symphysis
12 Superior vesical artery
13 Corpus cavernosum of penis
14 Prostate and prostatic part of urethra
15 Left seminal vesicle, cut in section
16 Bladder, with urethral openings marked with arrows
17 Left ureter
18 Left ductus (vas) deferens
19 Right ductus (vas) deferens
20 Inferior epigastric vessels
21 External iliac artery
22 External iliac vein
23 Internal iliac artery
24 Internal iliac vein
25 Ureter
26 Body of fifth lumbar vertebra
27 Fifth lumbar intervertebral disc
28 Promontory of sacrum
29 Sacrum
30 Coccyx
31 Cauda equina within sacral canal
32 Posterior wall of rectus sheath
33 Rectus abdominis
34 Rectovesical pouch

- The ureters (17, 25) conduct urine from the kidneys to the bladder (16) where it is stored until sensation of volume dictates expulsion via the single tube of the urethra (8), the extent of its full length seen here laying within the bisected shaft of the penis (7).
- The single prostate gland (14) and the paired seminal vesicles (15, left) are accessory secretory sex glands, which produce most of the volume of seminal fluid.
- The prostate gland (14), normally the size of a chestnut, lies just below the bladder (16) and opens into the urethra (8); the seminal vesicles (15, left) open into the ductus (vas) deferens (18, 19), which conduct sperm from the epididymis of each testis to the urethra (8) on ejaculation.
- The rectum (1) is the terminal part of the large intestine (colon) where faeces collect prior to defecation via the anus (4), the opening and closing of which is controlled by the muscles that form the external sphincter (3). The space between the rectum (1), prostate gland (14) and seminal vesicles (15, left) is known as the rectovesical pouch (34).

Superior

Anterior ⟷ Posterior

Inferior

Female pelvic viscera and vessels

Seen on the right side in a sagittal section, after removal of most of the peritoneum (serous membrane)

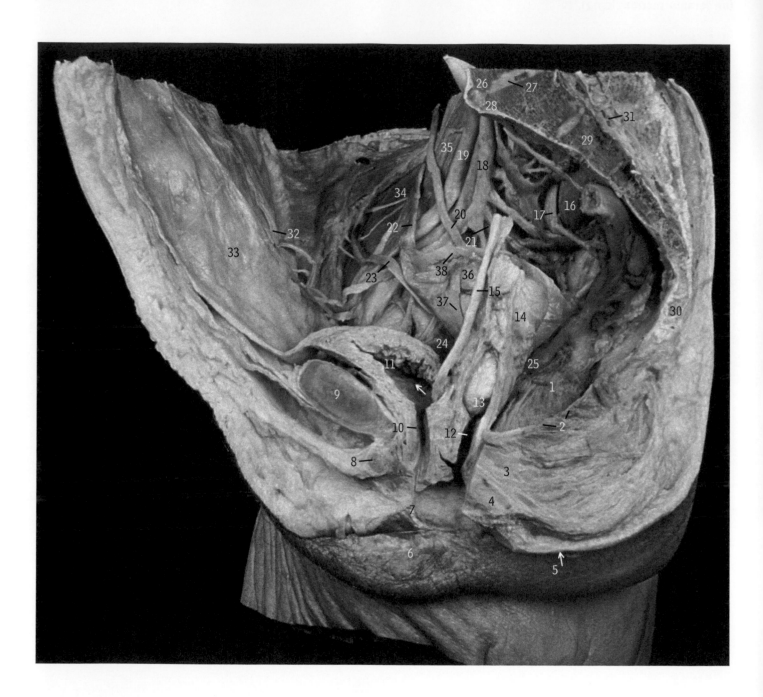

The section is mostly in the midline; small bowel, large bowel and much of the peritoneum (serous membrane) have been removed but the whole of the anal canal and the lower part of the left levator ani muscle have been preserved to show the external anal sphincter (as in the male section, p. 10).

1 Rectum
2 Cut edge of left levator ani
3 External anal sphincter covering anal canal
4 Perineal body (central perineal tendon)
5 Anus, above arrowhead
6 Labium majus
7 Labium minus
8 Clitoris
9 Pubic symphysis
10 Urethra, surrounded by sphincter urethrae
11 Bladder, arrow points to right ureter
12 Vagina
13 Cervix of uterus
14 Body of uterus
15 Left ureter
16 Piriformis
17 Anterior ramus of S1 nerve
18 External iliac vein
19 External iliac artery

20 Right ureter
21 Internal iliac vessels and branches
22 Ovarian vessels
23 Round ligament of uterus
24 Vesico-uterine pouch
25 Recto-uterine pouch (of Douglas)
26 Body of fifth lumbar vertebra
27 Fifth lumbar intervertebral disc
28 Promontory of sacrum
29 Sacrum
30 Coccyx
31 Sacral canal
32 Inferior epigastric vessels
33 Peritoneum overlying rectus abdominis [see 32–33, p. 10]
34 Iliacus
35 Psoas major
36 Right ovary
37 Right uterine (fallopian tube)
38 Right broad ligament

- The vagina (12) is the lower part of the female reproductive tract and lies in a central position between, anteriorly, the bladder (11) and, posteriorly, the rectum (1); superiorly, it connects the lower end of the uterus (the cervix) (13) with, inferiorly, the margin of the vaginal orifice and the labium majus (6) and labium minus (7).
- The urethra (10) in the female is much shorter in length, being only 4 cm, compared to that in the male, usually 18 cm; from the bladder it opens into the vaginal vestibule a few centimetres behind the clitoris (8). The space between the bladder (11) and the uterus (14) is known as the vesico-uterine pouch (24) and between the uterus (14) and the rectum (1) the recto-uterine pouch (of Douglas) (25).
- The body of the uterus (14) is pear shaped and normally lies over the bladder (11); from its sides the broad ligament (38, right) extends to the lateral walls of the pelvis. These help to keep the uterus in a central position.
- The ovaries (36, right) are suspended by part of the broad ligament (mesovarium) close to the lateral walls of the pelvis and are the main female reproductive organs; they produce cyclic steroid hormones as well as ovum (egg cells). The open ends of the uterine (fallopian) tubes (37, right) are positioned close to the ovaries, thus enabling discharged ova to freely enter them.

Superior

Anterior ← → Posterior

Inferior

Gluteal region *Sciatic nerve and other gluteal structures of the right side*

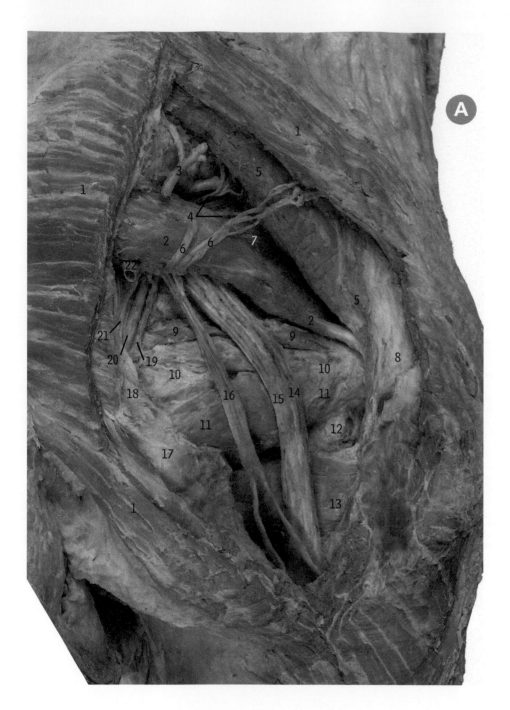

Most of gluteus maximus (1) has been removed (as have the veins that accompany arteries) to show the underlying structures, the most important of which is the sciatic nerve (14 and 15). The key to the region is the piriformis muscle (2): the superior gluteal artery (3) and nerve (4) emerge from the pelvis above piriformis, while all other structures leave the pelvis below piriformis. Apart from the sciatic nerve (14 and 15), these include the inferior gluteal nerve (6) and artery (22) and the posterior femoral cutaneous nerve (16).

1 Gluteus maximus
2 Piriformis
3 Superior gluteal artery
4 Superior gluteal nerve
5 Gluteus medius
6 Inferior gluteal nerve
7 Gluteus minimus
8 Greater trochanter of femur
9 Gemellus superior
10 Obturator internus
11 Gemellus inferior
12 Obturator externus
13 Quadratus femoris
14 Common fibular (*peroneal*) } part of sciatic nerve
15 Tibial
16 Posterior femoral cutaneous nerve
17 Ischial tuberosity
18 Sacrotuberous ligament
19 Nerve to obturator internus
20 Internal pudendal artery
21 Pudendal nerve
22 Inferior gluteal artery

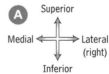

Superior / Medial / Lateral (right) / Inferior

Gluteal region *Surface features of the right gluteal region*

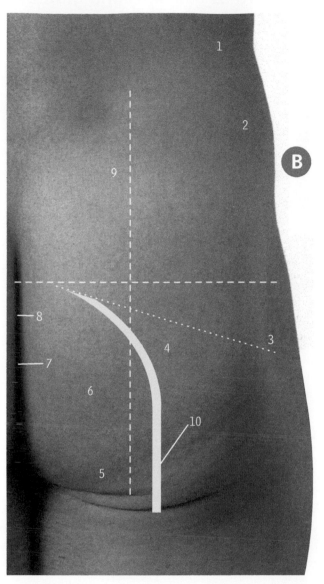

The interrupted lines divide the gluteal region into four quadrants. The surface marking of the lower border of piriformis (the dotted line) is on a line drawn from the midpoint between the posterior superior iliac spine (9) and the coccyx (7) to the top of the greater trochanter of the femur (3). From the midpoint of this line, a curved line (convex laterally) to midway between the ischial tuberosity (6) and the greater trochanter (3) indicates the course of the upper part of the sciatic nerve, indicated here in yellow.

- The superior gluteal nerve runs between gluteus medius and minimus and ends in tensor fasciae latae, supplying all three muscles.
- The inferior gluteal nerve passes straight back into gluteus maximus, supplying that muscle only.
- In the gluteal region the sciatic nerve is a flattened band about 1 cm broad. Its two parts (**A14** and **15**) are usually closely bound together in the gluteal region and the back of the thigh (p. 27, **B10**). In the popliteal fossa at the back of the knee (p. 32, **A**) they separate into the common fibular *(peroneal)* nerve, which supplies the front of the leg and dorsum of the foot, and the tibial nerve, which supplies the back of the leg and sole of the foot.

1 Iliac crest
2 Gluteus medius
3 Greater trochanter of femur
4 Gluteus maximus
5 Fold of buttock
6 Ischial tuberosity
7 Tip of coccyx
8 Natal cleft
9 Posterior superior iliac spine
10 Sciatic nerve

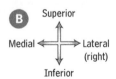

B   Superior
↑
Medial ◄——┼——► Lateral
↓   (right)
Inferior

Gluteal region

Left gluteal region and ischio-anal region, with gluteus maximus and gluteus medius cut through and portions reflected laterally

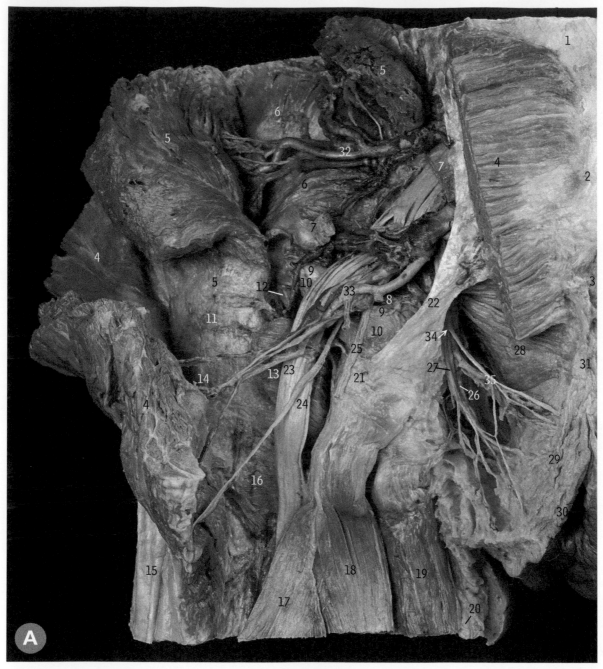

A   Superior ↑ / Lateral (left) ←→ Medial / Inferior ↓

1 Posterior layer of lumbar fascia overlying erector spinae	
2 Sacrum	
3 Coccyx	
4 Gluteus maximus	
5 Gluteus medius	
6 Gluteus minimus	
7 Piriformis	
8 Gemellus superior	
9 Obturator internus	
10 Gemellus inferior	
11 Greater trochanter of femur	
12 Obturator externus	

13 Quadratus femoris
14 Vastus lateralis
15 Iliotibial tract
16 Upper part of adductor magnus (adductor minimus)
17 Biceps femoris (long head)
18 Semitendinosus
19 Adductor magnus
20 Gracilis
21 Ischial tuberosity
22 Sacrotuberous ligament
23 Common fibular (*peroneal*) part of sciatic nerve

24 Tibial part of sciatic nerve
25 Posterior femoral cutaneous nerve
26 Internal pudendal artery
27 Pudendal nerve
28 Levator ani
29 External anal sphincter
30 Anal margin
31 Anococcygeal body
32 Superior gluteal artery, vein and nerve
33 Inferior gluteal artery, vein and nerve
34 Pudendal canal (arrowed)
35 Inferior rectal artery, vein and nerve

Gluteal region

Right gluteal region and ischio-anal region, with most of gluteus maximus removed

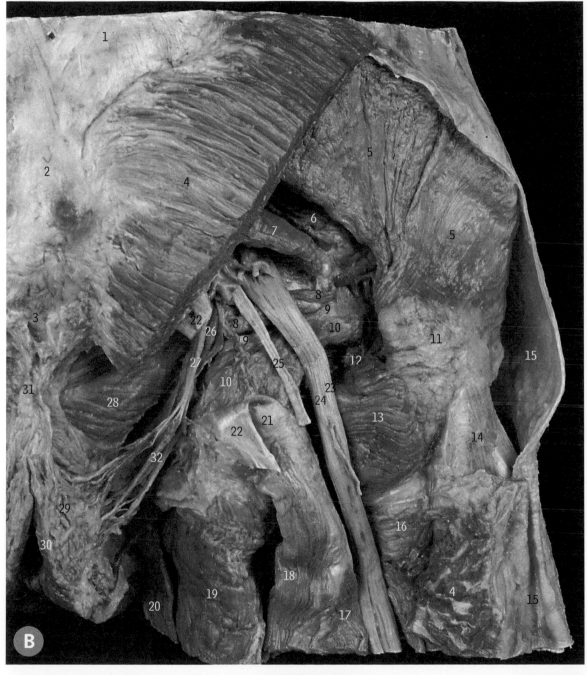

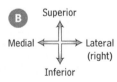

B   Superior

Medial ←——→ Lateral
(right)

Inferior

1 Posterior layer of lumbar fascia overlying erector spinae	**13** Quadratus femoris	**23** Common fibular (*peroneal*) part of sciatic nerve
2 Sacrum	**14** Vastus lateralis	**24** Tibial part of sciatic nerve
3 Coccyx	**15** Iliotibial tract	**25** Posterior femoral cutaneous nerve
4 Gluteus maximus	**16** Upper part of adductor magnus (adductor minimus)	**26** Internal pudendal artery
5 Gluteus medius	**17** Biceps femoris (long head)	**27** Pudendal nerve
6 Gluteus minimus	**18** Semitendinosus	**28** Levator ani
7 Piriformis	**19** Adductor magnus	**29** External anal sphincter
8 Gemellus superior	**20** Gracilis	**30** Anal margin
9 Obturator internus	**21** Ischial tuberosity	**31** Anococcygeal body
10 Gemellus inferior	**22** Sacrotuberous ligament cut and turned down	**32** Inferior rectal artery, vein and nerve
11 Greater trochanter of femur		
12 Obturator externus		

Hip joint *Left hip bone and femur, with sacrum and coccyx*

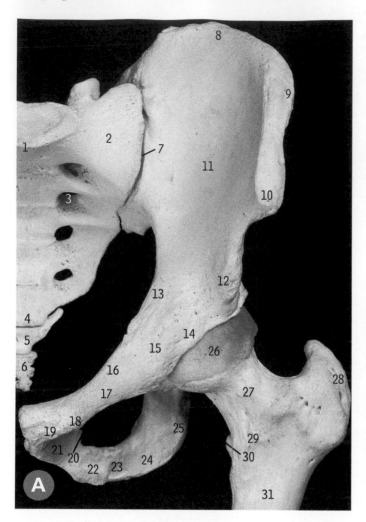

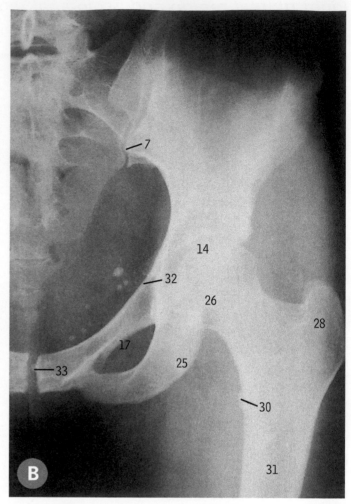

A **Left hip bone and femur, with sacrum and coccyx, from the front**

B **Radiograph. (The translucent areas are gas shadows in the large intestine.)**

1   Sacral promontory
2   Ala of sacrum
3   Second anterior sacral foramen, for anterior ramus of S2 nerve
4   Apex of sacrum
5   First coccygeal vertebra, with transverse process
6   Fused coccygeal vertebrae
7   Sacroiliac joint
8   Iliac crest, palpable throughout its whole length, and a possible site (like the sternum) for bone marrow biopsy
9   Tubercle of iliac crest
10 Anterior superior iliac spine, for inguinal ligament and sartorius
11 Iliac fossa, a term also applied to the lower lateral region of the anterior abdominal wall
12 Anterior inferior iliac spine, for part of rectus femoris
13 Arcuate line of ilium, forming part of the pelvic brim
14 Rim of acetabulum, the socket for the head of the femur (26)
15 Iliopubic eminence, site of union between ilium and superior ramus of the pubis (17)
16 Pectineal line (pecten) of pubis
17 Superior ramus of pubis

18 Pubic tubercle, a palpable landmark
19 Pubic crest, for rectus abdominis
20 Obturator foramen
21 Body of pubis
22 Inferior ramus of pubis
23 Site of union of pubic and ischial rami (22 and 24)
24 Ramus of ischium
25 Ischial tuberosity, best seen from behind (C16)
26 Head of femur
27 Neck, the part of the femur most commonly fractured
28 Greater trochanter. Gluteus medius and minimus are attached to its front and lateral side
29 Intertrochanteric line, for the capsule of the hip joint and not to be confused with the intertrochanteric crest on the back of the bone (C23)
30 Tip of lesser trochanter, best seen from behind (C25)
31 Shaft of femur
32 Ischial spine
33 Pubic symphysis

C Left hip bone and femur, with sacrum and coccyx, from behind

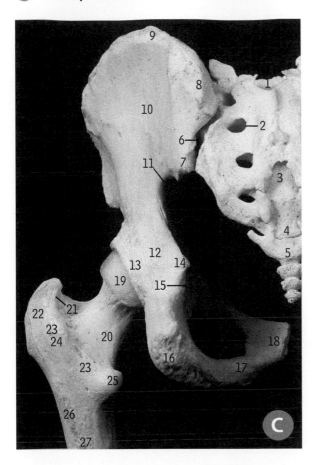

1 Sacral canal
2 Second posterior sacral foramen, for posterior ramus of S2 nerve
3 Sacral hiatus, the lower opening of the sacral canal and here unusually high
4 Apex of sacrum
5 First coccygeal vertebra, with below it the fused second to fourth coccygeal vertebrae
6 Sacroiliac joint
7 Posterior inferior iliac spine
8 Posterior superior iliac spine
9 Iliac crest
10 Ilium, outer surface
11 Greater sciatic notch
12 Site of fusion of ilium and ischium
13 Rim of acetabulum, the socket which receives the head of the femur (**19**)
14 Ischial spine, separating the greater and lesser sciatic notches (**11 and 15**)
15 Lesser sciatic notch
16 Ischial tuberosity, which bears the weight when sitting
17 Ramus of ischium joining inferior ramus of pubis
18 Body of pubis
19 Head of femur, making the hip joint with the acetabulum of the hip bone (**13**)
20 Neck, labeled along the site of attachment of the capsule of the hip joint, which does not extend as far as the intertrochanteric crest (**23**)
21 Trochanteric fossa for obturator externus
22 Greater tuberosity whose curved upper margin receives piriformis and obturator internus
23 Intertrochanteric crest
24 Quadrate tubercle, for quadratus femoris
25 Lesser trochanter, for psoas major with fibers from iliacus just below it
26 Gluteal tuberosity, receiving part of the attachment of gluteus maximus (the rest is attached to the fascia lata, the deep fascia of the thigh)
27 Shaft of femur

C
Superior
Lateral (left) ⟷ Medial
Inferior

D Left hip joint capsule (male), from the front, with all surrounding muscles removed except for obturator externus

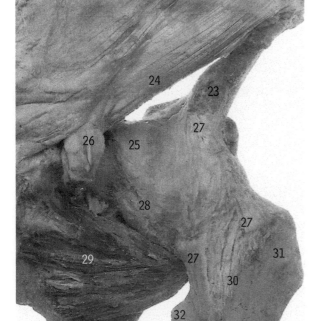

23 Anterior inferior iliac spine
24 Inguinal ligament
25 Iliopubic eminence
26 Spermatic cord
27 Iliofemoral ligament, like an inverted V, reinforcing and blending with the front of the capsule
28 Pubofemoral ligament, reinforcing and blending with the more medial part of the capsule
29 Obturator externus
30 Intertrochanteric line
31 Greater trochanter
32 Lesser trochanter

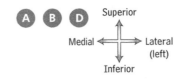

A B D
Superior
Medial ⟷ Lateral (left)
Inferior

Hip joint

Axial section through the left hip joint at the level of the last, fifth segment of the sacrum, from below

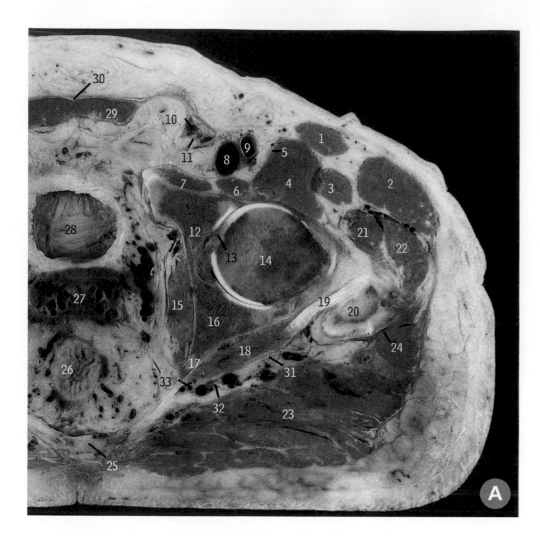

1 Sartorius
2 Tensor fasciae latae
3 Rectus femoris
4 Iliacus
5 Femoral nerve
6 Psoas major
7 Pectineus
8 Femoral vein
9 Femoral artery
10 Spermatic cord
11 Vas deferens
12 Acetabulum (pubic portion)
13 Ligamentum teres
14 Femoral head
15 Obturator internus
16 Ischium
17 Ischial spine
18 Gemellus superior
19 Obturator internus tendon
20 Greater trochanter
21 Gluteus minimus
22 Gluteus medius
23 Gluteus maximus
24 Trochanteric bursa
25 Sacrum fifth segment
26 Rectum
27 Seminal vesicle
28 Bladder
29 Rectus abdominis
30 Linea alba
31 Sciatic nerve
32 Inferior gluteal artery and vein
33 Pudendal nerve and internal pudendal artery and vein

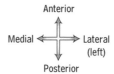

Anterior

Medial ⟵⟶ Lateral (left)

Posterior

Muscles producing movements at the hip joint consist of the following:

- **Flexion** (moving the thigh forward and upward toward the abdomen): psoas and iliacus, with rectus femoris, sartorius, tensor fasciae latae, pectineus, adductor longus and adductor brevis.
- **Extension** (moving the thigh backward): gluteus maximus, semimembranosus, semitendinosus, long head of biceps and ischial part of adductor magnus.
- **Abduction** (moving the thigh laterally away from the midline): gluteus medius, gluteus minimus, with tensor fasciae latae and piriformis.
- **Adduction** (moving the thigh medially toward the midline): adductor longus, adductor brevis, adductor magnus, pectineus, gracilis and quadratus femoris.

- **Medial rotation** (rotating the thigh inward in the long axis of the limb): anterior fibres of gluteus medius and gluteus minimus, with tensor fasciae latae. (Electromyography does not support the long-held view that psoas major is a medial rotator.)
- **Lateral rotation** (rotating the thigh outward in the long axis of the limb): obturator externus, obturator internus and gemelli, piriformis, quadratus femoris, gluteus maximus and sartorius.
- The coronal section of the joint in **C** demonstrates the thickness of the capsule (**C15**) but does not of course show the ligaments that reinforce the outside of the capsule (iliofemoral at the front, and pubofemoral and ischiofemoral below and behind).

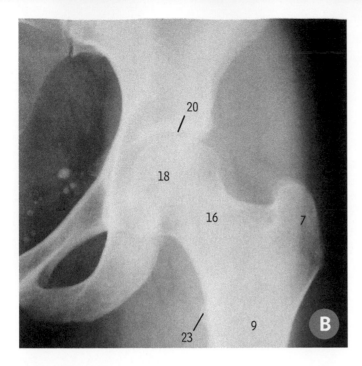

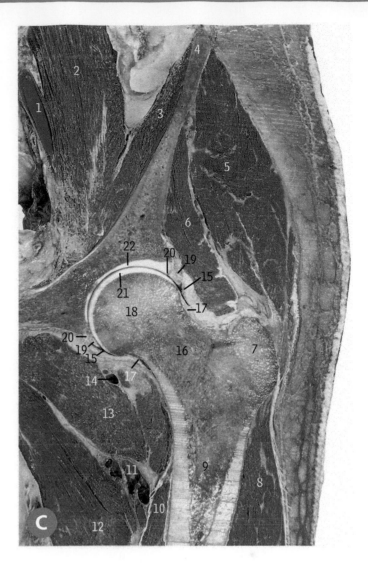

B Radiograph

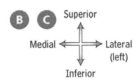

1   External iliac artery
2   Psoas major
3   Iliacus
4   Iliac crest
5   Gluteus medius
6   Gluteus minimus
7   Greater trochanter of femur
8   Vastus lateralis
9   Shaft of femur
10 Vastus medialis
11 Profunda femoris vessels
12 Adductor longus
13 Pectineus
14 Medial circumflex femoral
    vessels
15 Capsule of hip joint
16 Neck of femur
17 Zona orbicularis of capsule
18 Head of femur
19 Acetabular labrum
20 Rim of acetabulum
21 Hyaline cartilage of head of
    femur
22 Hyaline cartilage of
    acetabulum
23 Lesser trochanter of femur

B **C**   Superior

Medial ⬅➡ Lateral
           (left)

           Inferior

C Coronal section of the left hip joint, from the front

The head of the femur (18) sits in the hip bone's acetabulum (20), which is deepened at the periphery by the fibrous acetabular labrum (19). Note the hyaline cartilage on the joint surfaces (21 and 22), and the capsule (15) whose circular fibers (zona orbicularis, 17) keep it close to the neck of the femur (16). Gluteus medius (5) and gluteus minimus (6) converge on to the greater trochanter (7), and below the head and neck of the femur (18 and 16), the tendon of psoas major (2) and some muscle fibres of iliacus (3) are passing backward to reach the lesser trochanter on the back of the bone. Compare major features in the section with the radiograph.

Thigh, knee and leg

2

Thigh

Front of the right thigh (female), superficial structures of the femoral triangle

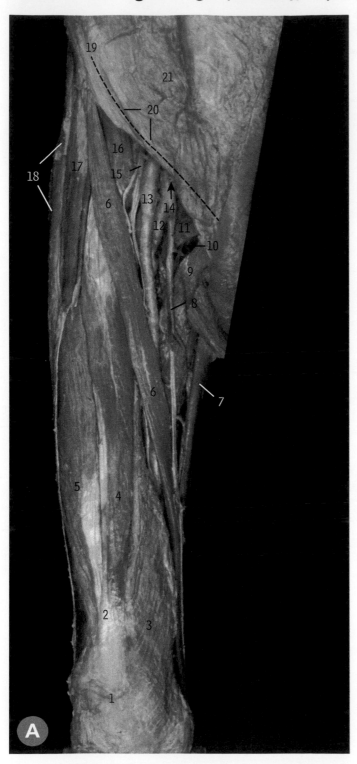

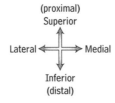

1 Patella
2 Tendon of quadriceps femoris
3 Vastus medialis
4 Rectus femoris
5 Vastus lateralis
6 Sartorius
7 Gracilis
8 Great saphenous vein
9 Adductor longus
10 Adductor brevis
11 Pectineus
12 Femoral vein
13 Femoral artery
14 Femoral canal (arrowed)
15 Femoral nerve
16 Iliacus
17 Tensor fascia latae
18 Iliotibial tract
19 Anterior superior iliac spine
20 Position of inguinal ligament
21 External oblique aponeurosis

The inguinal ligament (20):
- Attaches (like a bow string) taught between the anterior superior iliac spine (superolaterally) and the pubic tubercle (inferomedially) of that side of the pelvis
- Has an adult length between 12–14 cm
- Inclines at an angle between 35–40 degrees

The femoral triangle:
- **Boundaries** are the inguinal ligament (**20**), medial border of sartorius (**6**) and medial border of adductor longus (**9**)
- Is shaped like a gutter
- From lateral to medial, contains the key structures, femoral nerve (**15**), artery (**13**), vein (**12**) and canal (**14**)

The femoral canal (14):
- Opens into the peritoneal cavity via the femoral ring behind the inguinal ligament
- Is approximately 4 cm in length in adults
- Forms the most medial compartment of the femoral sheath
- Gives passage for lymphatic channels from the lower limb into the pelvis
- By providing space, allows the femoral vein to expand and thus increase venous drainage to the lower limb

The femoral pulse:
- Can be located and palpated below the inguinal ligament and midway between the anterior superior iliac spine and the pubic symphysis (p. 26 **B**)

(proximal)
Superior

Lateral ◄────► Medial

Inferior
(distal)

Thigh

Back of the right thigh (female) and gluteal region

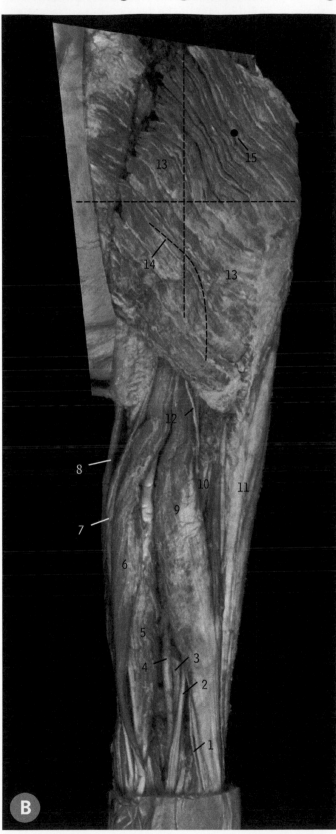

1. Common fibular (peroneal) nerve
2. Tibial nerve
3. Popliteal vein
4. Popliteal artery
5. Semitendinosus
6. Semimembranosus
7. Adductor magnus
8. Gracilis
9. Long head } of biceps femoris
10. Short head }
11. Iliotibial tract
12. Posterior cutaneous femoral nerve
13. Gluteus maximus
14. Position of sciatic nerve
15. Site for intramuscular injection (the upper outer quadrant)

Gluteal intramuscular injection
The bulky gluteus maximus muscle (13) with gluteus medius underneath is a possible site for *intramuscular injections,* but it is of course absolutely vital to choose the correct position for injection in order to avoid damaging the sciatic nerve (14).

The proper site is usually described as **the upper outer quadrant** of the gluteal region (15).

In estimating the four quadrants by vertical and horizontal lines through the midpoint of the region, it must be remembered that the most **upper** boundary of the region is the *iliac crest,* not the most prominent part of the bulge of the buttock or a suntanned bikini line, which are both far too low.

Only by choosing the properly defined quadrant can injury to the sciatic nerve be avoided. (See p. 15 for detailed description.)

The needle should enter either gluteus maximus or the adjacent part of gluteus medius.

The popliteal fossa:
- Is a diamond-shaped area at the back of the knee

Upper boundaries are:
- Lateral side, biceps femoris (with common fibular (peroneal) nerve behind it)
- Medial side, semimembranosus (with tendon of semitendinosus behind it)

Lower boundaries are:
- Laterally, the lateral head of gastrocnemius and plantaris
- Medially, the medial head of gastrocnemius

Key structures within the fossa are:
- Superficial to deep, the tibial nerve, popliteal vein and popliteal artery (See also p. 38.)

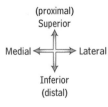

(proximal)
Superior

Medial ⟵⟶ Lateral

Inferior
(distal)

Thigh *Front of the right upper thigh (female)*

Part of the fascia lata (deep fascia of the thigh, 14) has been removed to display the femoral vessels and nerve and the adjacent muscles. The femoral nerve (21), artery (20), vein (18) and canal (17) lie in that order from lateral to medial beneath the inguinal ligament (19). The great saphenous vein (12) passes through the saphenous opening (16) in the fascia lata to enter the femoral vein (18); a number of smaller veins enter the great saphenous just before it joins the femoral.

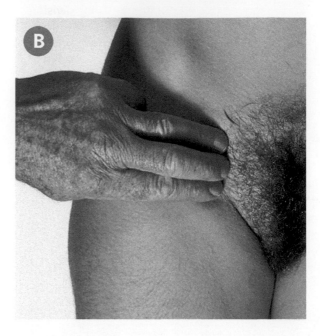

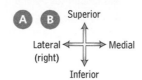

Ⓐ Inguinal and femoral regions, in the female

Ⓑ Palpation of femoral pulse

Ⓐ Ⓑ Superior ↑ Lateral ←→ Medial (right) ↓ Inferior

- The femoral pulse can be felt midway between the anterior superior iliac spine and the midline pubic symphysis (the midinguinal point or femoral point).

1 Anterior superior iliac spine
2 External oblique aponeurosis
3 Cut edge of rectus sheath
4 Rectus abdominis
5 Superficial epigastric vein
6 Superficial inguinal ring
7 Round ligament of uterus
8 Mons pubis
9 Gracilis
10 Adductor longus
11 Pectineus
12 Great saphenous vein
13 Superficial external pudendal vessels
14 Fascia lata
15 Accessory saphenous vein
16 Lower edge of saphenous opening
17 Position of femoral canal
18 Femoral vein
19 Inguinal ligament
20 Femoral artery
21 Femoral nerve
22 Medial
23 Intermediate } femoral cutaneous nerve
24 Sartorius
25 Superficial circumflex iliac vessels
26 Fascia lata overlying tensor fasciae latae

- Various superficial veins (**5, 13, 15, 25**) run into the great saphenous vein (**12**); this helps to distinguish the great saphenous from the femoral vein (**18**), which superficially at this level receives only the great saphenous itself. See p. 76 for further details of the great saphenous vein.
- Although arising at the *front* of the thigh, the profunda femoris artery (**C24**) is the main supply to muscles on the *back* of the thigh as well as those on the front.
- The adductor canal, which is triangular in cross section, is bounded in front by sartorius (**24**), laterally by vastus medialis, and behind by adductor longus (**10**) (above) and adductor magnus (below). The contents of the adductor canal are the femoral artery and vein (**20** and **18**), the saphenous nerve (**C25**) and the nerve to vastus medialis (**C20**).

Thigh *Front of the right upper thigh (male)*

In this deeper dissection, the removal of part of sartorius (3) displays the profunda femoris artery (24). The femoral artery (9) passes in front of adductor longus (18); the profunda (24) passes behind it. Separation of the adjacent borders of pectineus (13) and adductor longus (18) allows the anterior division of the obturator nerve (15) to be seen in front of adductor brevis (17). The medial circumflex femoral artery (12) disappears backward between pectineus

(13) and the tendon of psoas (hidden behind the uppermost part of the femoral artery (upper 9). The lateral circumflex femoral artery (11, which often arises directly from the femoral artery, as here, and not from the profunda) courses laterally and supplies adjacent muscles. Branches of the femoral nerve (8) include the saphenous nerve (25), which will run as far as the medial side of the foot.

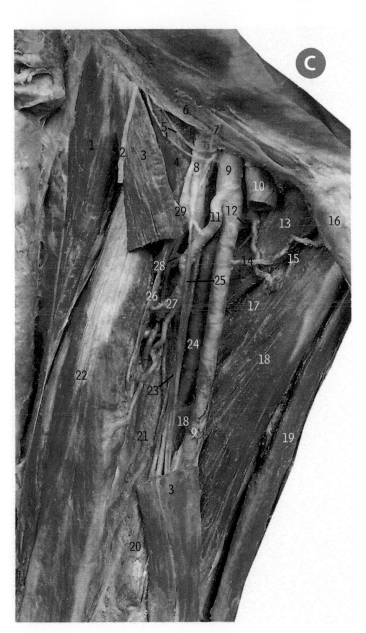

1 Tensor fasciae latae
2 Lateral femoral cutaneous nerve
3 Sartorius
4 Iliacus
5 Superficial circumflex iliac artery (double)
6 Inguinal ligament
7 Superficial epigastric artery
8 Femoral nerve
9 Femoral artery
10 Femoral vein
11 Lateral circumflex femoral artery
12 Medial circumflex femoral artery
13 Pectineus
14 Superficial external pudendal artery
15 Anterior branch of obturator nerve
16 Spermatic cord
17 Adductor brevis
18 Adductor longus
19 Gracilis
20 Vastus medialis
21 Vastus intermedius
22 Rectus femoris
23 Nerve to vastus medialis
24 Profunda femoris artery
25 Saphenous nerve
26 Nerve to rectus femoris
27 Descending ⎫
28 Transverse ⎬ branch of lateral circumflex femoral
29 Ascending ⎭ artery

Superior

Lateral ⟷ Medial
(right)

Inferior

C Femoral vessels and nerve, in the male

Thigh *Lower right thigh, medial side*

The lower part of sartorius (3) has been displaced medially to open up the lower part of the adductor canal and expose the femoral artery (4) passing through the opening in adductor magnus (6) to enter the popliteal fossa behind the knee and become the popliteal artery.

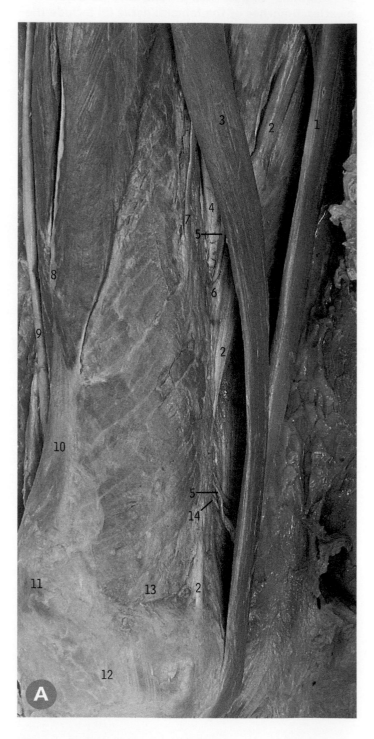

1 Gracilis
2 Adductor magnus
3 Sartorius
4 Femoral artery
5 Saphenous nerve
6 Opening in adductor magnus
7 Vastus medialis and nerve
8 Rectus femoris
9 Iliotibial tract
10 Quadriceps tendon
11 Patella
12 Medial patellar retinaculum
13 Lowest (horizontal) fibres of vastus medialis
14 Saphenous branch of descending genicular artery

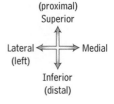

(proximal)
Superior

Lateral ⟵ ⟶ Medial
(left)

Inferior
(distal)

A From the front and medial side

Thigh *Axial section through lower right thigh*

The section is viewed as when looking upward from knee to hip. The three vastus muscles (1, 3, 5) envelop the femur (2) at the front and sides, and rectus femoris (4) at this level is narrow and is becoming tendinous. The femoral vessels (20) are between vastus medialis (1) and adductor magnus (12), approaching the adductor magnus opening (13), and the profunda femoris vessels (11) lie close to the back of the femur (2). The sciatic nerve (10) is deeply placed between biceps (8, 9) laterally and semimembranosus (14) and semitendinosus (15) medially.

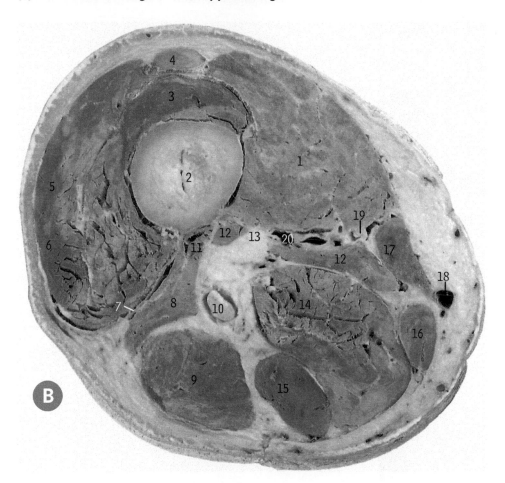

1 Vastus medialis
2 Femur
3 Vastus intermedius
4 Rectus femoris
5 Vastus lateralis
6 Iliotibial tract
7 Lateral intermuscular septum
8 Short head } of biceps
9 Long head
10 Sciatic nerve
11 Profunda femoris vessels
12 Adductor magnus
13 Opening in adductor magnus
14 Semimembranosus
15 Semitendinosus
16 Gracilis
17 Sartorius
18 Great saphenous vein
19 Saphenous nerve
20 Femoral vessels

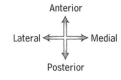

Anterior

Lateral ⟵⟶ Medial

Posterior

B Axial section at the level of the opening in adductor magnus

- The muscles commonly called the hamstrings span both the hip and knee joints: they arise from the ischial tuberosity and run to the upper end of the tibia and fibula, and consist of semitendinosus, semimembranosus, and the long head of biceps. The short head of biceps is not a hamstring; although it joins the long head, it arises from the back of the femur and hence does not span the hip joint. Semitendinosus is named from the long tendon at its lower end. Semimembranosus is named from the broad tendinous origin at its upper end.

Knee joint *Left knee joint*

Flexion of the knee, as in B, exposes a much larger area of the femoral condyles (4, 7) than is seen in extension (as in A and C). In B the medial and lateral menisci (18, 22) lie between the condyles of the femur and tibia (4, 9; 7, 12), with the anterior cruciate ligament (19) passing backward and laterally from the upper surface of the tibia to the medial surface of the lateral condyle of the femur. Compare the MR image in C with the dissection in B.

In D the joint has been opened up by cutting through the quadriceps muscle (26) and the patellar ligament (30) and turning laterally the large flap which includes the patella (28), in order to show the joint cavity from the front and the margins of the suprapatellar bursa (27), which is in direct continuity with the cavity of the knee joint.

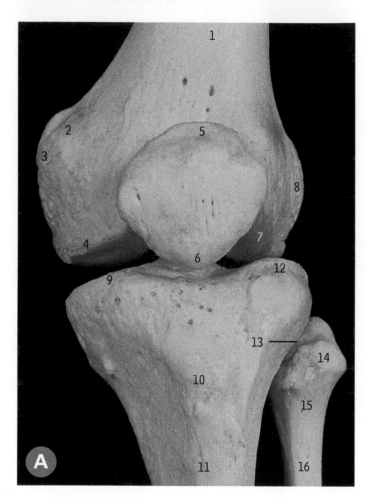

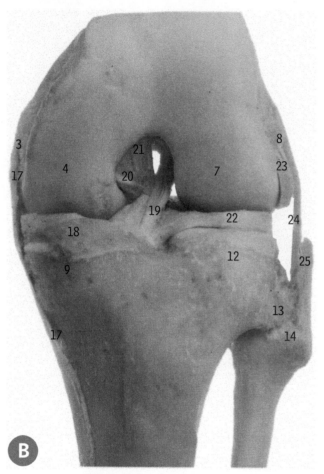

Ⓐ **Bones, with the knee joint in extension, from the front**

Ⓑ **Bones and ligaments, with the knee joint in flexion and the patella removed, from the front**

- The **lateral ligament (B24**, properly called the fibular collateral ligament) is a rounded cord about 5 cm long, passing from the lateral epicondyle of the femur (**B8**) to the head of the fibula (**B14**).
- The **medial ligament (B17**, properly called the tibial collateral ligament) is a broad flat band about 12 cm long passing from the medial epicondyle of the femur (**B3**) to the medial side of the medial condyle of the tibia (**B9**) and to an extensive area of the medial surface below the condyle. At the side it fuses with the medial meniscus (**B18**; see also p. 33, **B18** and **19**); the lateral ligament (**B24**) does not fuse with the lateral meniscus (**B22**), to which the tendon of popliteus has an attachment (p. 33, **C28**).
- For notes on the cruciate ligaments and menisci, see p. 32.

1 Shaft of femur
2 Adductor tubercle
3 Medial epicondyle
4 Medial condyle
5 Base of patella
6 Apex of patella
7 Lateral condyle
8 Lateral epicondyle
9 Medial condyle of tibia
10 Tibial tuberosity
11 Shaft
12 Lateral condyle
13 Superior tibiofibular joint (with capsule in B)
14 Head ⎤
15 Neck ⎬ of fibula
16 Shaft ⎦

17 Medial ligament
18 Medial meniscus
19 Anterior cruciate ligament
20 Anterior meniscofemoral ligament
21 Posterior cruciate ligament
22 Lateral meniscus
23 Popliteus tendon
24 Lateral ligament
25 Biceps tendon
26 Quadriceps femoris
27 Margins of suprapatellar bursa
28 Posterior surface of patella
29 Infrapatellar fat pad
30 Patellar ligament
31 Deep infrapatellar bursa

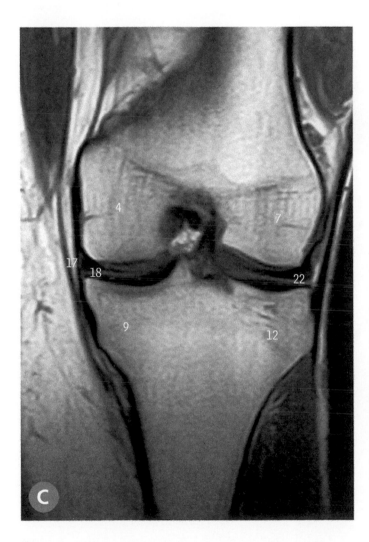

C Coronal magnetic resonance image (MRI)

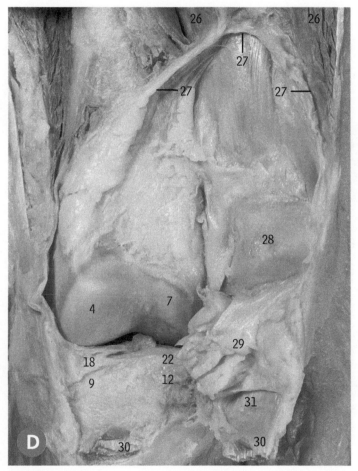

D Opened up from the front, with the knee joint in extension and the patella turned laterally

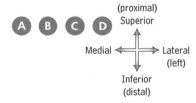

(proximal)
Superior

Medial ⟷ Lateral
(left)

Inferior
(distal)

Knee joint *Left knee joint*

The joint in B is partly flexed, showing less of the articular surfaces of the femoral condyles (4, 6) than in A. In B the posterior cruciate ligament (20) spills over onto the uppermost part of the posterior surface of the tibia. The attachment of the medial meniscus (19) to the medial ligament (18) is clearly seen; the lateral meniscus (23) has no attachment to the lateral ligament (24) but gives rise to the posterior meniscofemoral ligament (22), which lies on the surface of the posterior cruciate ligament (20), here obscuring the anterior meniscofemoral ligament (27).

The view in C demonstrates the shapes of the medial and lateral menisci (19, 23), the tibial attachments of the anterior and posterior cruciate ligaments (21, 20) and the anterior and posterior meniscofemoral ligaments (27, 22), which pass respectively in front of and behind the posterior cruciate ligament (20).

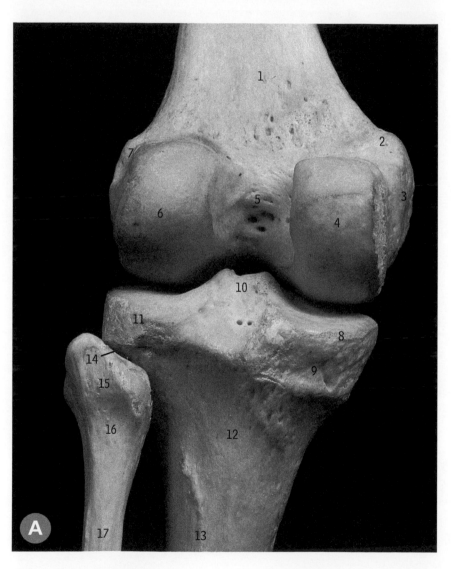

 1 Popliteal surface of femur
 2 Adductor tubercle
 3 Medial epicondyle
 4 Medial condyle
 5 Intercondylar fossa
 6 Lateral condyle
 7 Lateral epicondyle
 8 Medial condyle of tibia
 9 Groove for semimembranosus insertion
10 Intercondylar eminence
11 Lateral condyle of tibia
12 Popliteal surface of tibia
13 Soleal line
14 Superior tibiofibular joint (with capsule in B)
15 Head   ⎫
16 Neck   ⎬ of fibula
17 Shaft   ⎭
18 Medial ligament
19 Medial meniscus
20 Posterior cruciate ligament
21 Anterior cruciate ligament
22 Posterior meniscofemoral ligament
23 Lateral meniscus (with marker under medial margin in C)
24 Lateral ligament
25 Popliteus tendon
26 Biceps tendon
27 Anterior meniscofemoral ligament
28 Attachment of popliteus to lateral meniscus

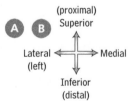

A Bones, from behind

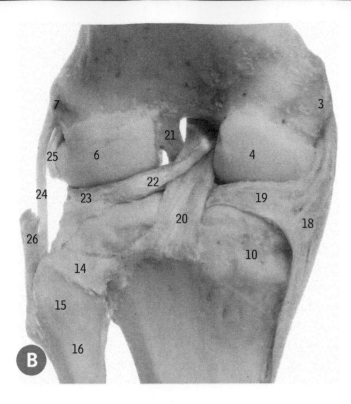

B Ligaments, from behind

- The cruciate ligaments are named from their attachments to the tibia.
- The anterior cruciate ligament (**C21**), from the front of the upper surface of the tibia, passes upward, backward and laterally to become attached to the medial side of the lateral condyle of the femur (p. 30, **B19**).
- The posterior cruciate ligament (**C20**), from the back of the upper surface and the very top of the posterior surface of the tibia, passes upward, forward and medially to become attached to the lateral side of the medial condyle of the femur (p. 30, **B21**).
- The anterior and posterior meniscofemoral ligaments (**C27, C22**) arise from the back of the lateral meniscus and run upward and forward like a two-pronged fork embracing the posterior cruciate ligament (**C20**) at its front and back and fusing with it.
- The C-shaped fibrocartilaginous menisci (**C19** and **C23**) are attached by their ends (the horns of the menisci) to the intercondylar area of the upper surface of the tibia.
- Muscles producing movements at the knee joint include the following:
  Flexion (bending the leg backwards): semimembranosus, semitendinosus, biceps, gracilis, sartorius, gastrocnemius and popliteus.
  Extension (straightening the flexed knee): vastus medialis, vastus intermedius, vastus lateralis, rectus femoris, and tensor fasciae latae and gluteus maximus acting via the iliotibial tract.
  Medial rotation *of the flexed leg* (rotating the leg medially in the long axis of the leg): semimembranosus, semitendinosus, gracilis, sartorius and popliteus.
  Lateral rotation *of the flexed leg* (rotating the leg laterally in the long axis of the leg): biceps.
- Because of the shape of the articulating surfaces and the tension in the ligaments, there is some medial rotation of the femur on the tibia toward the end of extension (assuming the tibia to be fixed); this is the so-called 'locking of the knee joint'. To begin flexion, popliteus 'unlocks' the joint by causing some lateral rotation of the femur on the tibia (assuming the tibia to be fixed); the other flexors can then carry on the movement.

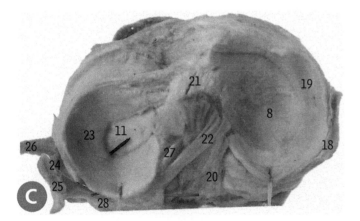

C Upper surface of tibia with ligaments, from above

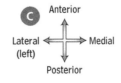

Anterior

Lateral ⟷ Medial
(left)

Posterior

Knee joint

Coronal section through the left knee joint (male), from the front

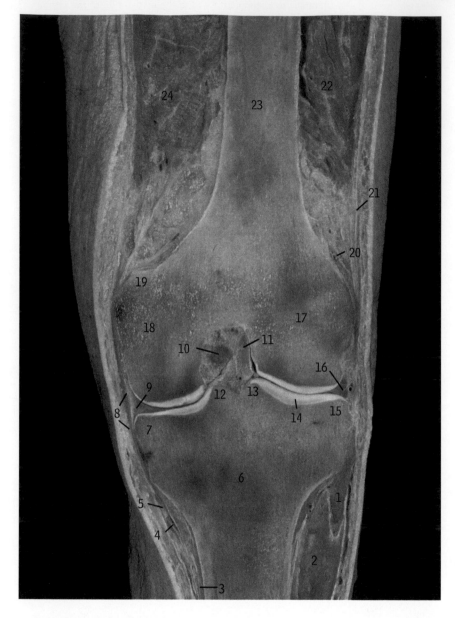

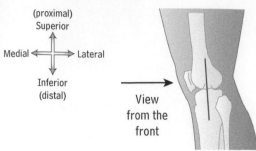

(proximal)
Superior

Medial ⟷ Lateral

Inferior
(distal)

View
from the
front

1 Extensor digitorum longus
2 Tibialis anterior
3 Popliteus (most medial fibres)
4 Gracilis (tendon)
5 Sartorius (tendon)
6 Tibia
7 Medial condyle (plateau) of tibia
8 Tibial (medial) collateral ligament
9 Medial meniscus
10 Posterior ⎫ cruciate ligament
11 Anterior ⎭
12 Medial ⎫ intercondylar tubercle of tibia
13 Lateral ⎭
14 Articular cartilage
15 Lateral condyle (plateau) of tibia
16 Lateral meniscus
17 Lateral ⎫ condyle of femur
18 Medial ⎭
19 Adductor tubercle of femur
20 Superior genicular artery
21 Fascia lata
22 Vastus lateralis
23 Shaft of femur
24 Vastus medialis

The knee joint:
- Is a hinge joint
- Is the largest synovial joint in the body
- Is formed by the unions of the two condyles of the femur
  (**17, 18**) and the two condyles of the tibia (**7, 15**) along with
  the patella, which articulates solely with the condyles of the
  femur
- Provides movements of flexion, extension and small degree of
  rotation

The tibial (medial) collateral ligament (8):
- Runs from the medial epicondyle of the femur to the upper part
  of the medial surface of the tibia
- Is a broad, flat, band-like structure approximately 12 cm in length
  (See p. 30 for a more detailed description.)

The fibular (lateral) collateral ligament:
- Passes from the lateral epicondyle of the femur to the apex of the
  head of the fibula
- Is a rounded structure approximately 5 cm in length
  (See p. 30 for a more detailed description.)

The anterior and posterior cruciate ligaments (10, 11):
- Are main factors that hold the femur and tibia together within
  the knee joint
- Are strong bands which cross each other in the shape of an 'X'
  when viewed from the side as in a sagittal section
- Pass from the inside surfaces of the femoral condyles to the
  central intercondylar area on the upper surface of the tibia
- Are covered by synovial membrane at their fronts and sides but
  not at the back
  (See p. 33 for a more detailed description.)

Knee joint

Sagittal section I through the left knee joint (female), from the left

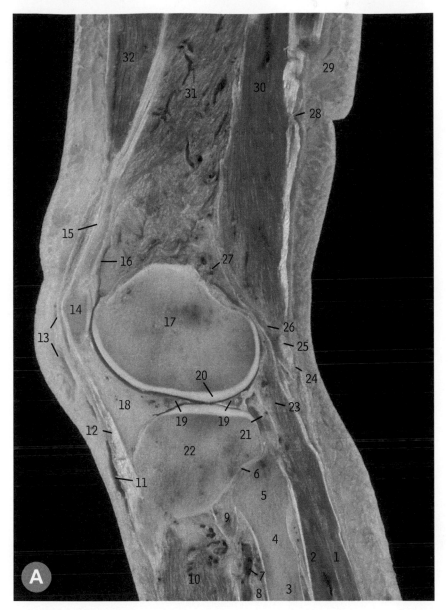

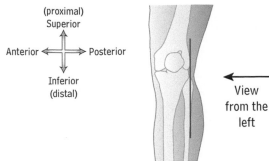

(proximal)
Superior

Anterior ⟷ Posterior

Inferior
(distal)

View
from the
left

1 Gastrocnemius lateral head
2 Soleus
3 Shaft ⎫
4 Neck ⎬ of fibula
5 Head ⎭
6 Superior tibiofibular joint
7 Anterior tibial artery and vein
8 Interosseous membrane
9 Tibialis posterior
10 Tibialis anterior
11 Infrapatellar bursa
12 Patellar ligament
13 Prepatellar bursa
14 Patella
15 Tendon of quadriceps femoris
16 Suprapatellar bursa
17 Lateral condyle of femur
18 Infrapatellar fat pad extending into infrapatellar fold
19 Lateral meniscus
20 Articular cartilage
21 Popliteus (tendon)
22 Lateral condyle (plateau) of tibia
23 Plantaris
24 Lateral cutaneous nerve of calf
25 Common fibular (peroneal) nerve
26 Fibrous capsule of knee joint
27 Lateral superior geniculate artery
28 Deep ⎫
   ⎬ fascia
29 Superficial ⎭
30 Biceps femoris
31 Vastus intermedius
32 Vastus lateralis

The fibrous capsule (26):
- Covers all aspects of the knee joint except at the front where its place is taken by the patella and patellar ligament
- Is lined by a synovial membrane

The infrapatellar fat pad (18):
- Pushes the synovial membrane backwards below the patella to fill up the gap between the femoral and tibial epicondyles

The medial and lateral (19) meniscus:
- Are main factors that hold the femur and tibia together outside the capsule of the knee joint
- Lay on top of the articular surfaces of the tibia
- Are C-shaped in appearance when viewed from above

- Are composed of fibrocartilage, which is thick at the periphery and very thin toward the centre
- Are not covered by synovial membrane
- Are attached by the 'horns' of their 'C' shape to the intercondylar area of the tibia near to the cruciate ligaments
- The medial meniscus is also firmly attached to the medial cruciate ligament
- The lateral meniscus is not attached to the lateral cruciate ligament
- Fill up space between the curved femoral condyles and flat articular surfaces of the tibia and help spread synovial fluid over the bones
- Act as shock absorbers and bear over half the weight transmitted across the joint

Knee joint

Sagittal section II through the left knee joint (female), from the left

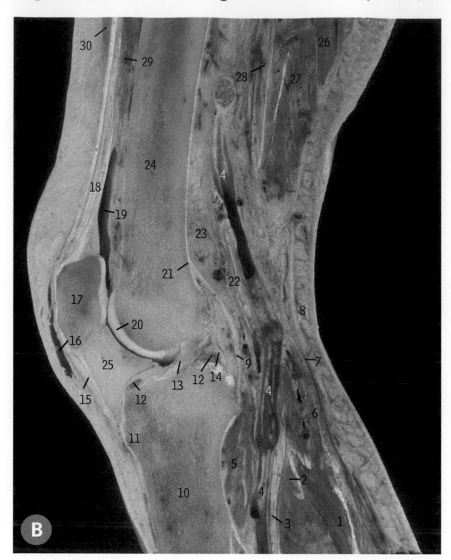

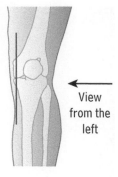

View from the left

(proximal)
Superior

Anterior ←→ Posterior

Inferior
(distal)

1 Soleus	**17** Patella
2 Plantaris (tendon)	**18** Tendon of quadriceps femoris
3 Tibial nerve	**19** Suprapatellar bursa
4 Popliteal vein	**20** Articular cartilage
5 Popliteus	**21** Popliteal surface of femur
6 Gastrocnemius	**22** Popliteal artery
7 Deep ⎱ fascia	**23** Popliteal pad of fat
8 Superficial ⎰	**24** Shaft of femur
9 Fibrous capsule of knee joint	**25** Infrapatellar fat pad extending into
10 Shaft ⎱ of tibia	infrapatellar fold
11 Tuberosity ⎰	**26** Semitendinosus
12 Medial meniscus	**27** Semimembranosus
13 Anterior ⎱ cruciate ligament	**28** Sciatic nerve
14 Posterior ⎰	**29** Vastus intermedius
15 Patellar ligament	**30** Rectus femoris
16 Prepatellar bursa	

The patella (17):
- Is situated within the tendon of quadriceps femoris (**18**)
- Is the largest sesamoid bone in the body
- Is held at a constant distance from the upper surface of the tibia by the patellar ligament (**15**)
- Slides over the femoral condyles as the knee joint bends
- Never comes into contact with the tibia

The suprapatellar bursa (19):
- Communicates with the synovial cavity of the knee joint
- Extends behind the tendon of quadriceps femoris (**18**) for three finger-breadths above the upper border of the patella
- May fill with excessive synovial fluid when the knee joint is injured resulting in 'fluid on the knee' that may be drained by needle aspiration

Knee joint

Sagittal section III through the left knee joint (female), from the left

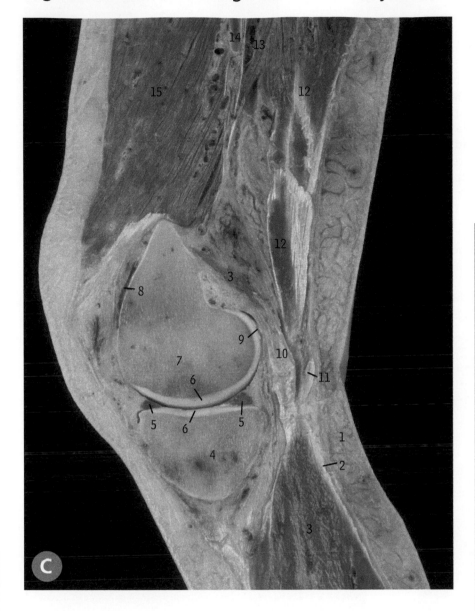

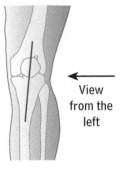

View from the left

The articular cartilage (6):
- Formed on the distal ends of the femoral and tibial condyles, is hyaline cartilage
- Is lubricated by synovial fluid within the knee joint cavity that is normally no more in quantity than a mere 0.5 ml

Principle muscles producing knee joint movement are:
Flexion (bending)
- Hamstrings, gastrocnemius and popliteus
Extension (straightening)
- Quadriceps femoris
Medial rotation
- of tibia, when semi-flexed: semimembranosus and semitendinosus
Lateral rotation
- of tibia, when semi-flexed: biceps femoris
(See p. 33 for more detailed description.)

Arterial supply to the knee joint is from the:
- Descending genicular branches of the femoral artery
- Middle and inferior genicular branches of the popliteal artery
- Anterior and posterior branches of the anterior tibial artery
- Circumflex fibular artery
- Descending branch of the lateral circumflex femoral artery

Nerve supply to the knee joint is from the:
- Obturator nerve
- Femoral nerve
- Tibial nerve
- Common fibular (peroneal) nerve

1 Superficial } fascia
2 Deep
3 Gastrocnemius medial head
4 Medial condyle (plateau) of tibia
5 Medial meniscus
6 Articular cartilage
7 Medial condyle of femur
8 Suprapatellar bursa
9 Fibrous capsule of knee joint
10 Tendon of medial head of gastrocnemius
11 Tendon of semitendinosus
12 Semimembranosus
13 Adductor magnus
14 Femoral artery
15 Vastus medialis

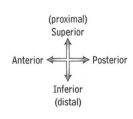

(proximal) Superior
Anterior ⟷ Posterior
Inferior (distal)

Knee joint

Popliteal fossa and back of the knee

In A the fascia that forms the roof of the fossa and the fat within it have been removed. At the upper part of the fossa, biceps (10) is on the lateral side with the common fibular (*peroneal*) nerve (9) at its posterior border, and semimembranosus (3) with semitendinosus (4) overlying it are on the medial side. At the lower part of the fossa, the medial head of gastrocnemius (15) is on the medial side, whereas on the lateral side plantaris (11) lies just above the lateral head of gastrocnemius (12). Of the principal structures within the fossa, the tibial nerve (7) is the most superficial, with the popliteal vein (6) behind it and the popliteal artery (5) deep to the vein.

In the lateral view in B, the ridge formed by the iliotibial tract (18) lies above (anterior to) the tendon of biceps (10), at the lateral boundary of the popliteal fossa (25). Below the head of the fibula (24) the common fibular (*peroneal*) nerve (9) is palpable and can be rolled against the neck of the bone.

1 Sartorius
2 Gracilis
3 Semimembranosus
4 Semitendinosus
5 Popliteal artery
6 Popliteal vein
7 Tibial nerve
8 Lateral cutaneous nerve of calf
9 Common fibular (*peroneal*) nerve
10 Biceps
11 Plantaris
12 Lateral head of gastrocnemius
13 Small saphenous vein (double)
14 Sural nerve
15 Medial head of gastrocnemius
16 Nerve to medial head } of gastrocnemius
17 Nerve to lateral head
18 Iliotibial tract
19 Patella
20 Margin of lateral condyle of femur
21 Patellar ligament
22 Tuberosity of tibia
23 Margin of lateral condyle of tibia
24 Head of fibula
25 Popliteal fossa

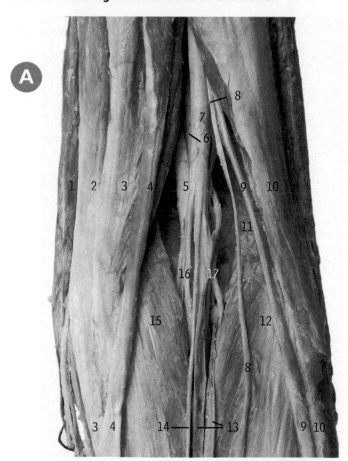

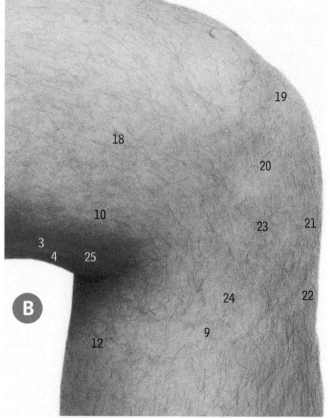

A Right popliteal fossa

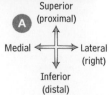

Superior (proximal)

Medial ⟷ Lateral (right)

Inferior (distal)

B Surface landmarks of the flexed right knee, from the lateral side

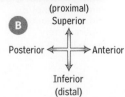

(proximal) Superior

Posterior ⟷ Anterior

Inferior (distal)

Knee joint

Popliteal fossa and back of the knee

Most of gastrocnemius, soleus and other muscles have been removed to display popliteus (6) and the posterior surface of the knee joint capsule (13), which is reinforced by the tendinous fibers of semimembranosus (11) that form the oblique popliteal ligament (12).

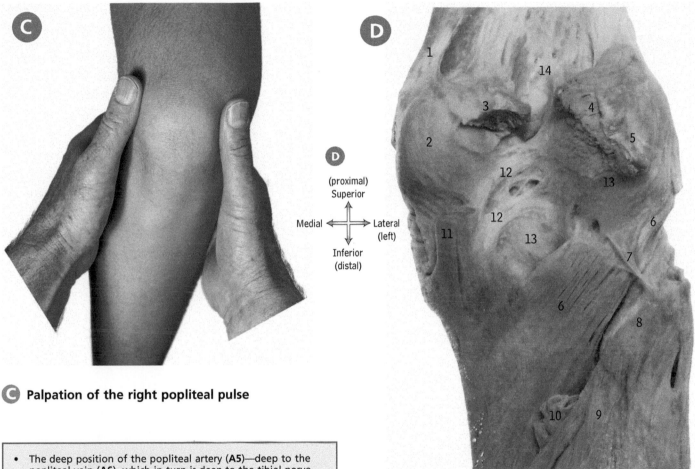

(proximal)
Superior

Medial ⟷ Lateral
(left)

Inferior
(distal)

C Palpation of the right popliteal pulse

D Right popliteus muscle and knee joint capsule, from behind

- The deep position of the popliteal artery (**A5**)—deep to the popliteal vein (**A6**), which in turn is deep to the tibial nerve (**A7**)—makes feeling the popliteal pulse difficult. It is best felt from the front, grasping the sides of the knee with both hands, placing the thumbs beside the patella and pressing the tips of the fingers deeply into the midline of the fossa.

- The slender arcuate popliteal ligament (**D7**) arches over popliteus (**D6**) as it enters the joint capsule to reach the lateral side of the lateral condyle of the femur.

 1 Adductor magnus
 2 Capsule overlying medial condyle of femur
 3 Medial head of gastrocnemius
 4 Plantaris
 5 Lateral head of gastrocnemius
 6 Popliteus
 7 Arcuate popliteal ligament
 8 Head of fibula
 9 Soleus
10 Popliteal vessels and tibial nerve
11 Semimembranosus
12 Oblique popliteal ligament
13 Capsule of knee joint
14 Popliteal surface of femur

Leg and foot survey

Muscles and superficial vessels and nerves of the left leg and foot

Skin, subcutaneous tissue and most of the deep fascia have been removed, and different aspects of the same specimen are shown. Lateral to the medial (subcutaneous) surface (A2) and anterior border of the tibia is the largest muscle of the front of the leg, tibialis anterior (A6, C6), which becomes tendinous in the lower part of the leg and has the tendons of extensor hallucis longus (A7) and extensor digitorum longus (A8) lateral to it. On the medial side the bulk of gastrocnemius (A3, B3) and the underlying soleus (A4) overlie the flexor muscles whose tendons pass behind the medial malleolus (B9)—tibialis posterior (B19),

flexor digitorum longus (B18) and flexor hallucis longus (B16), in that order from front to back. On the lateral side, fibularis (peroneus) longus (C23) largely overlies fibularis *(peroneus)* brevis (C25); their tendons pass behind the lateral malleolus (C10). At the back gastrocnemius (D3) has been detached at its upper end to show the underlying soleus (E4), which in turn has been detached with plantaris (E31) in F to display the underlying flexor muscle—tibialis posterior (F19), the deepest muscle, which is overlapped by flexor hallucis longus (F16) on the lateral side and flexor digitorum longus (F18) on the medial side.

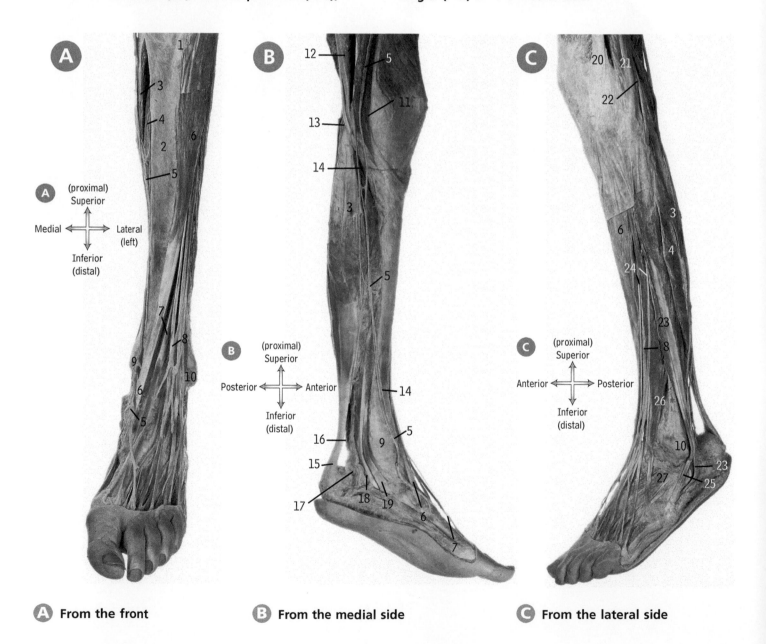

A From the front

B From the medial side

C From the lateral side

1 Patellar ligament (lower edge)
2 Medial surface of tibia
3 Gastrocnemius
4 Soleus
5 Great saphenous vein
6 Tibialis anterior
7 Extensor hallucis longus
8 Extensor digitorum longus
9 Medial malleolus
10 Lateral malleolus
11 Sartorius
12 Gracilis
13 Semitendinosus
14 Saphenous nerve
15 Tendo calcaneus
16 Flexor hallucis longus
17 Tibial nerve and posterior tibial vessels

18 Flexor digitorum longus
19 Tibialis posterior
20 Iliotibial tract
21 Biceps femoris
22 Common fibular *(peroneal)* nerve
23 Fibularis *(peroneus)* longus
24 Superficial fibular *(peroneal)* nerve
25 Fibularis *(peroneus)* brevis
26 Fibularis *(peroneus)* tertius
27 Extensor digitorum brevis
28 Semimembranosus
29 Small saphenous vein
30 Sural nerve
31 Plantaris
32 Tibial nerve
33 Popliteal vein overlying artery
34 Fascia over popliteus

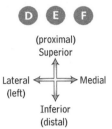

(proximal)
Superior

Lateral ←——→ Medial
(left)

Inferior
(distal)

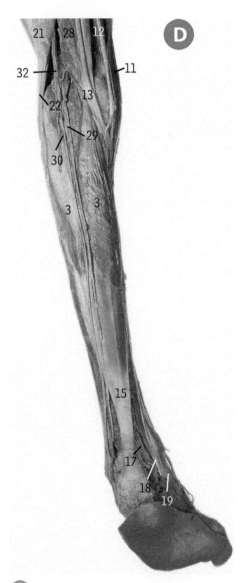

D **From behind**

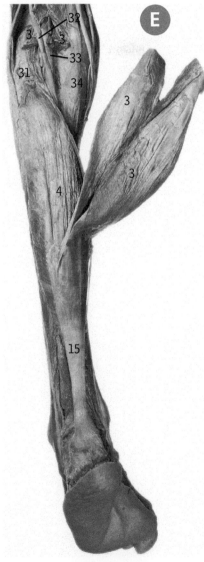

E **From behind, with gastrocnemius detached**

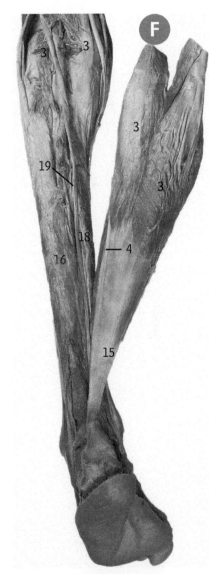

F **From behind, with gastrocnemius, plantaris and soleus detached**

Foot

3

Surface landmarks of the foot *Surface landmarks of the left foot*

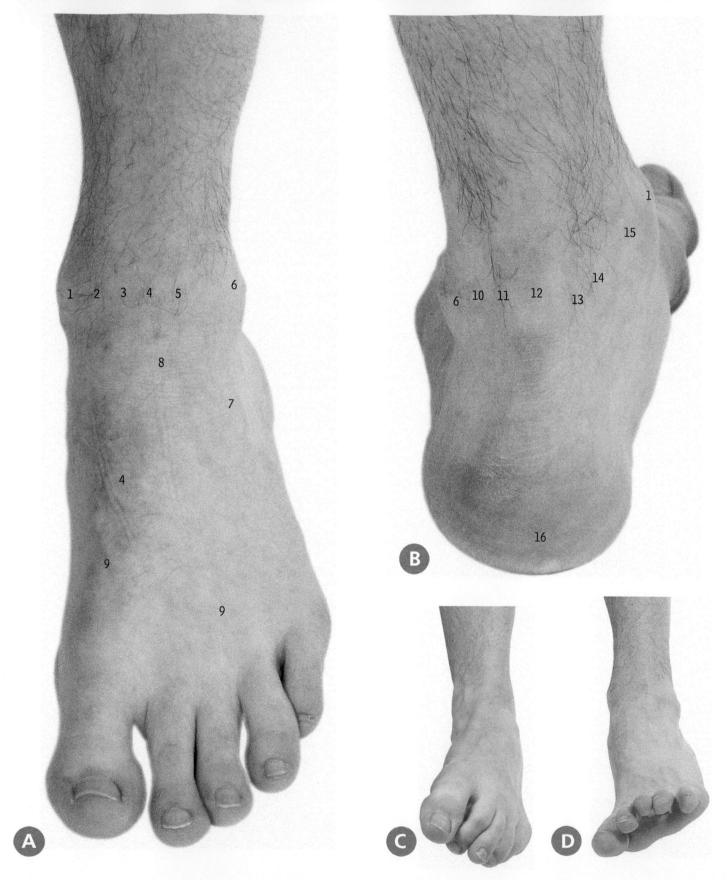

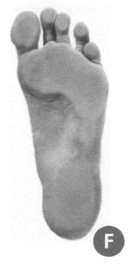

1 Medial malleolus
2 Great saphenous vein and saphenous nerve
3 Tibialis anterior
4 Extensor hallucis longus
5 Extensor digitorum longus
6 Lateral malleolus
7 Extensor digitorum brevis
8 Dorsalis pedis artery
9 Dorsal venous arch
10 Fibularis (*peroneus*) longus and brevis
11 Small saphenous vein and sural nerve
12 Tendo calcaneus
13 Flexor hallucis longus
14 Posterior tibial artery and tibial nerve
15 Flexor digitorum longus and tibialis posterior
16 Tuberosity of calcaneus
17 Sesamoid bones under head of first metatarsal
18 Base of first metatarsal
19 Head of fifth metatarsal
20 Tuberosity of base of fifth metatarsal
21 Tuberosity of navicular

F

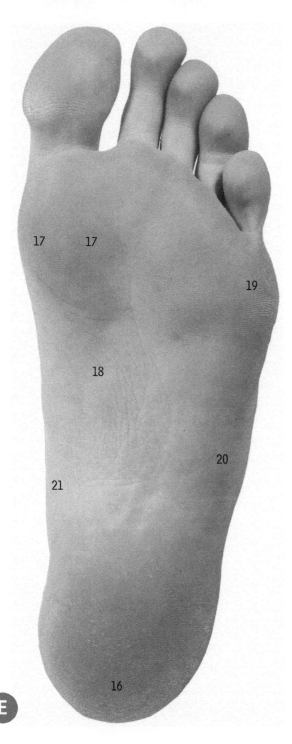

E

Definitions of movements are as follows:
- **Extension:** from the Latin for straightening out, but as far as the ankle and foot are concerned it means bending the foot and/or toes upwards, which also known as dorsiflexion.
- **Flexion:** from the Latin for bending. In the ankle and foot it means bending the foot and/or toes downwards, which is also known as plantarflexion.
- **Abduction:** from the Latin for moving away. In the foot it means spreading the toes apart (the corresponding movement of the fingers Is much more extensive).
- **Adduction:** from the Latin for moving toward. In the foot it means drawing the toes together.
- **Inversion:** from the Latin for turning in—turning the foot so that the sole faces more inwards (medially).
- **Eversion:** from the Latin for turning out—moving the foot so that the sole faces more outwards (laterally) (a more limited movement than inversion).

For further details see pp. 85 and 107.

A From the front and above (dorsal surface, dorsum)

B From behind

C From the front, in inversion

D From the front, in eversion with abduction of toes

E From below (plantar surface, sole)

F Imprint of sole when weight-bearing (viewed through a glass plate)

Surface landmarks of the foot *Surface landmarks of the left foot*

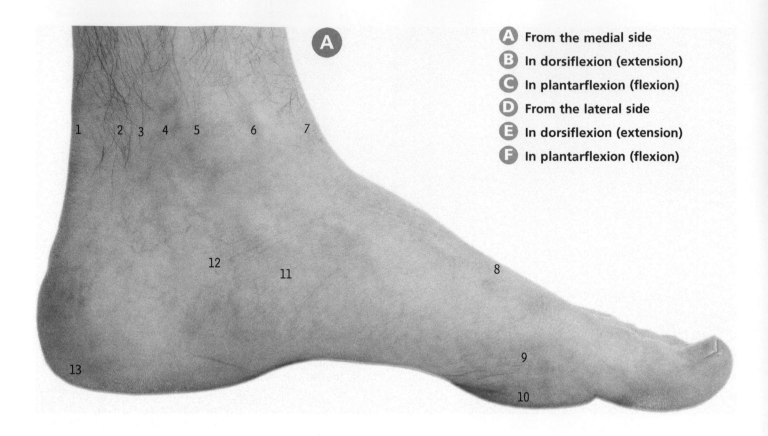

A From the medial side
B In dorsiflexion (extension)
C In plantarflexion (flexion)
D From the lateral side
E In dorsiflexion (extension)
F In plantarflexion (flexion)

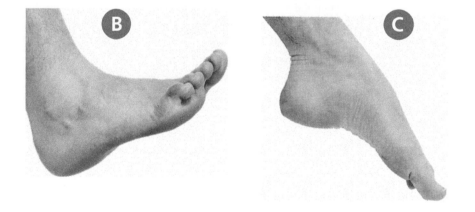

1   Tendo calcaneus
2   Flexor hallucis longus
3   Posterior tibial artery and tibial nerve
4   Flexor digitorum longus and tibialis posterior
5   Medial malleolus
6   Great saphenous vein and saphenous nerve
7   Tibialis anterior
8   Extensor hallucis longus
9   Head of first metatarsal
10 Sesamoid bone
11 Tuberosity of navicular
12 Sustentaculum tali
13 Tuberosity of calcaneus
14 Small saphenous vein and sural nerve
15 Fibularis *(peroneus)* longus and brevis
16 Lateral malleolus
17 Extensor digitorum brevis
18 Extensor digitorum longus
19 Tuberosity of base of fifth metatarsal
20 Head of fifth metatarsal

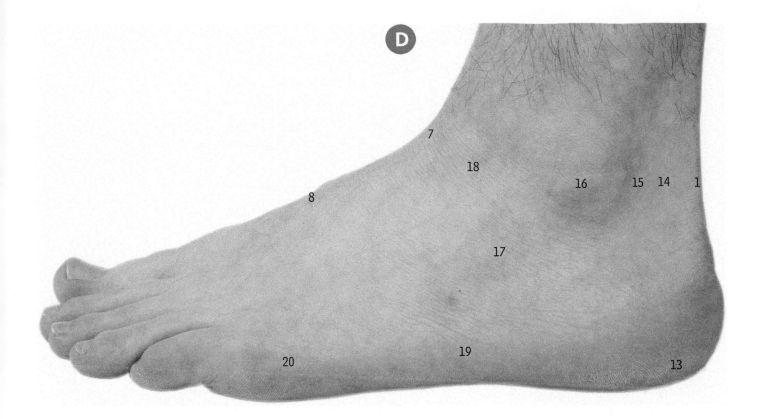

D

7

18

16   15   14   1

8

17

19

20   13

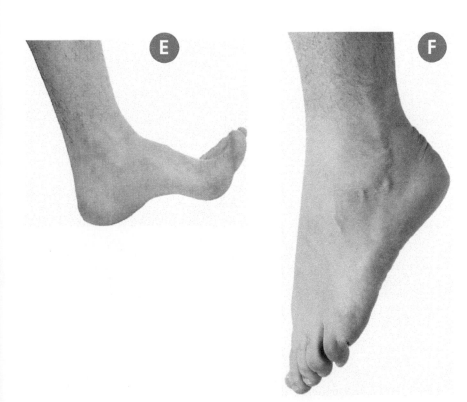

E

F

- Pulsation in the dorsalis pedis artery (p. 80, **14**) is normally palpable between the tendons of extensor hallucis longus (**8**) and extensor digitorum longus (**18**), on a line from the midpoint between the medial and lateral malleoli to the proximal end of the first intermetatarsal space. However, the artery is absent in about 12% of feet (see p. 85).
- Pulsation in the posterior tibial artery (**3**) is normally palpable behind the medial malleolus (**5**), 2.5 cm in front of the medial border of the tendo calcaneus.
- The sustentaculum tali (**12**) is palpable about 2.5 cm below the tip of the medial malleolus (**5**).

Skeleton of the foot *Bones of the left foot, from above*

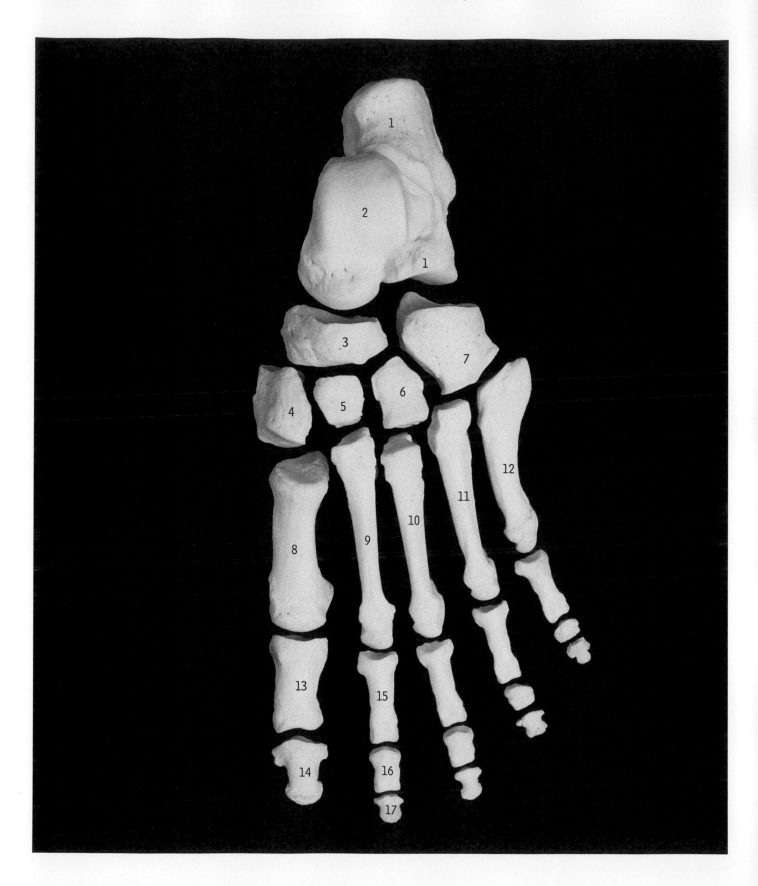

The talus and calcaneus remain articulated with each other but the remainder have been disarticulated.

1 Calcaneus
2 Talus
3 Navicular
4 Medial cuneiform
5 Intermediate cuneiform
6 Lateral cuneiform
7 Cuboid
8 First metatarsal
9 Second metatarsal
10 Third metatarsal
11 Fourth metatarsal
12 Fifth metatarsal
13 Proximal phalanx ⎫
14 Distal phalanx ⎬ of great toe
15 Proximal phalanx ⎫
16 Middle phalanx ⎬ of second toe
17 Distal phalanx ⎭

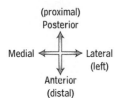

(proximal)
Posterior

Medial ←——→ Lateral
              (left)

Anterior
(distal)

- **Bones of the tarsus**
  Calcaneus
  Talus
  Navicular bone
  Cuboid bone
  Medial, intermediate and lateral cuneiform bones
- **Bones of the metatarsus**
  First to fifth metatarsal bones, numbered from medial to lateral
- **Bones of the toes or digits**
  Phalanges—a proximal and a distal phalanx for the great toe; proximal, middle and distal phalanges for each of the second to fifth toes
- The **hindfoot** consists of the talus and calcaneus.
- The **midfoot** consists of the navicular, cuboid and cuneiform bones.
- The **forefoot** consists of the metatarsal bones and phalanges.
- **Sesamoid bones**—two always present in the tendons of flexor hallucis brevis. For others see pp. 50, 52.
- **Origin and meaning of some names associated with the foot** are as follows (some older names for bones are given in parentheses):

Tibia:	Latin for a flute or pipe; when held upside down, the shin bone has a fanciful resemblance to this wind instrument.
Fibula:	Latin for a pin or skewer; the long thin bone of the leg. Adjective fibular or peroneal, which is from the Greek for pin (see the last note on p. 3).
Tarsus:	Greek for a wicker frame, in the basic framework for the back of the foot.
Metatarsus:	Greek for beyond the tarsus; the forepart of the foot.
Talus: (astragalus)	Latin (Greek) for one of a set of dice; viewed from above the main part of the talus has a rather square appearance.
Calcaneus: (os calcis, calcaneum)	From the Greek for heel; the heel bone.
Navicular: (scaphoid)	Latin (Greek) for boat-shaped; the navicular bone roughly resembles a saucer-shaped coracle.
Cuboid:	Greek for cube-shaped.
Cuneiform:	Latin for wedge-shaped.
Phalanx:	Greek for a row of soldiers; a row of bones in the toes. Plural phalanges.
Sesamoid:	Greek for shaped like a sesame seed.
Digitus:	Latin for finger or toe. Digiti and digitorum are the genitive singular and genitive plural—of the toe(s).
Hallux:	Latin for the great toe. Hallucis is the genitive singular—of the great toe.
Dorsum:	Latin for back; the upper surface of the foot. Adjective dorsal.
Plantar:	Adjective from planta, Latin for the sole of the foot.

Skeleton of the foot *Articulated bones of the left foot*

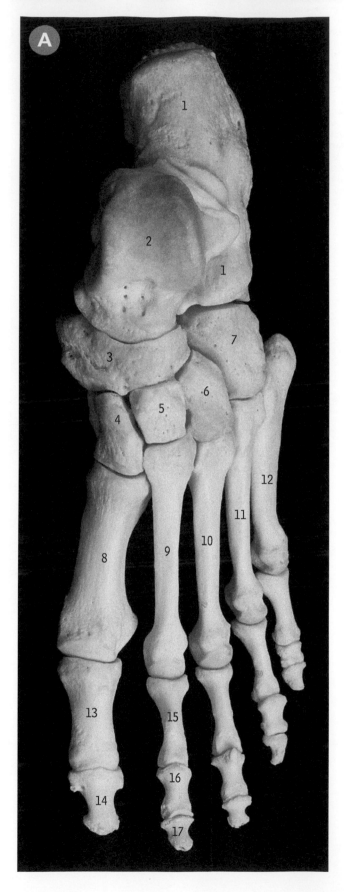

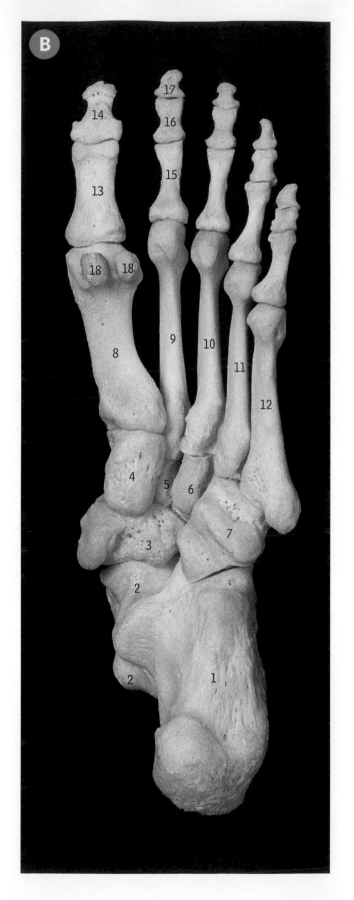

1 Calcaneus
2 Talus
3 Navicular
4 Medial cuneiform
5 Intermediate cuneiform
6 Lateral cuneiform
7 Cuboid
8 First metatarsal
9 Second metatarsal
10 Third metatarsal
11 Fourth metatarsal
12 Fifth metatarsal
13 Proximal phalanx } of great toe
14 Distal phalanx
15 Proximal phalanx
16 Middle phalanx } of second toe
17 Distal phalanx
18 Sesamoid bones

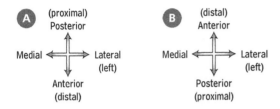

A From above (dorsal surface)

B From below (plantar surface)

Ossification of foot bones
All the tarsal bones are ossified from one primary center: calcaneus at the third fetal month, talus at the sixth fetal month, cuboid just before or just after birth, lateral cuneiform at 1 year, medial cuneiform at 2 years, intermediate cuneiform and navicular at 3 years.

The calcaneus is the only tarsal bone to have a secondary center: a thin plate of bone on the posterior surface, appearing at about 7 years and fusing during puberty.

The metatarsal bones and phalanges have primary centers for their shafts at the second to fourth fetal months, and one secondary center at the base of the first metatarsal and bases of all the phalanges but at the heads of the other metatarsals. These begin to ossify at 2 to 6 years and fuse at about 18 years.

All dates given are subject to considerable variation, and ossification tends to occur earlier in females.
- During the preparation of dried bones, the hyaline cartilage on articulating surfaces is lost, so that when rearticulating bones an exact fit is not possible. The thickness of the cartilage on joint surface is best appreciated in sections of bones, as on pp. 20, 21 and 100–112.
- The **talus** (2) is the uppermost foot bone, forming the ankle joint with the tibia and fibula. For details see pp. 58, 67.
- The **calcaneus** (1) is the most posterior and the largest foot bone, forming the heel. For details see pp. 68, 69.
- The **navicular bone** (3) lies in front of the talus, on the medial side of the foot. For details see p. 70.
- The **cuboid bone** (7) lies in front of the calcaneus, on the lateral side of the foot. For details see p. 70.
- The **three cuneiform bones**—medial, intermediate and lateral (4, 5 and 6)—lie in front of the navicular bone. For details see p. 71.
- The first, second and third **metatarsal bones** (8, 9 and 10) are in front of the three cuneiforms, and the fourth and fifth metatarsal bones (11 and 12) are in front of the cuboid bone. For details see pp. 72, 73.
- The **phalanges** (13–17) are the bones of the toes. Each proximal phalanx articulates with the head of a metatarsal bone. Each phalanx has a base (at the proximal end), body and head (at the distal end). The body is convex on the dorsal (upper) surface, and concave on the plantar surface. See pp. 48, 56.

Skeleton of the foot

Attachments of muscles and major ligaments to the bones of the left foot

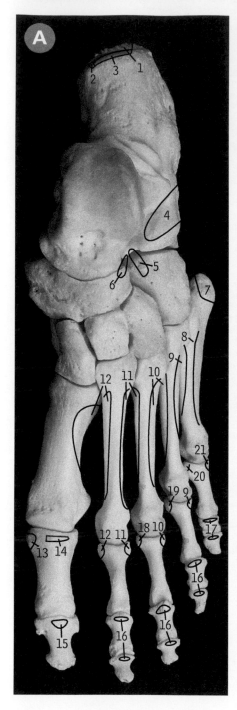

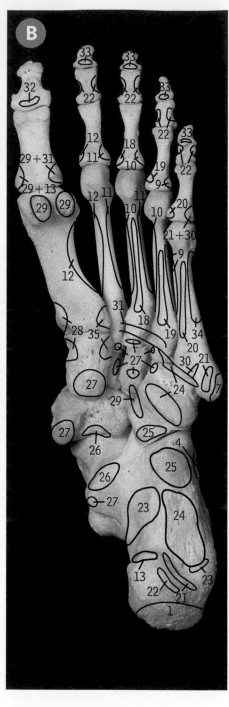

1 Tendo calcaneus
2 Plantaris
3 Area for bursa
4 Extensor digitorum brevis
5 Calcaneocuboid part ⎫ of bifurcate
6 Calcaneonavicular part ⎭ ligament
7 Fibularis (peroneus) brevis
8 Fibularis (peroneus) tertius
9 Fourth ⎫
10 Third ⎬ dorsal interosseus
11 Second ⎪
12 First ⎭
13 Abductor hallucis
14 Extensor hallucis brevis
15 Extensor hallucis longus
16 Extensor digitorum longus and brevis
17 Extensor digitorum longus
18 First ⎫
19 Second ⎬ plantar interosseus
20 Third ⎭
21 Abductor digiti minimi
22 Flexor digitorum brevis
23 Quadratus plantae
24 Long plantar ligament
25 Plantar calcaneocuboid (short plantar)
   ligament
26 Plantar calcaneonavicular (spring) ligament
27 Tibialis posterior
28 Tibialis anterior
29 Flexor hallucis brevis
30 Flexor digiti minimi brevis
31 Adductor hallucis
32 Flexor hallucis longus
33 Flexor digitorum longus
34 Opponens digiti minimi (occasional part
   of 30)
35 Fibularis (peroneus) longus

A From above (dorsal surface)   **B** From below (plantar surface)

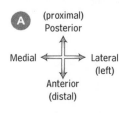

A   (proximal)
     Posterior

Medial ⟷ Lateral
              (left)

     Anterior
     (distal)

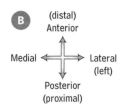

B   (distal)
     Anterior

Medial ⟷ Lateral
              (left)

     Posterior
     (proximal)

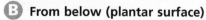

Sesamoid and accessory bones

Sesamoid bones

The patella is by far the largest sesamoid bone in the lower limb, and its close association with tendons and a bony joint (the knee) gives a conceptual focus as to the function of sesamoid bones.

In the foot:
- They usually vary in shape and size but in general are ovoid and normally only a few millimeters in diameter (p. 50, **B18**).
- They are not always ossified but may consist of fibrous tissue or cartilage, or a combination of all three.
- They are usually found embedded in tendons at the point where the tendons angle acutely around bony surfaces to their point of insertion (p. 100, **16** and p. 101, **33**).
- Sesamoids have articular cartilage on the surface which is in direct relationship to the bone that they are proximate to.

Although not proved, it is thought that sesamoid bones protect tendons from wear and, by their strategic position to joints, alter the angle of insertion of a tendon into bone and thus provides a greater mechanical advantage to the joint.

Accessory bones

Bones within the human body gradually begin to form during the early developmental phases of the fetus by the initial formation of central areas of ossification within the cartilaginous and membranous skeleton. These ossified areas continue to grow, unite and eventually form solid adult bones, some during late childhood and some as late as early adulthood.

On occasions, however, the centres of ossification fail to fuse completely, often at the ends of bones, and thus a separate (accessory or supernumerary) bone is formed.

The foot is a common place for accessory bones to form, and there are common sites for them to occur. It is important to be aware of their possible presence because on a radiographic image they can be easily mistaken for a fractured bone or 'chip'.

Common accessory bones in the foot are:
- **Dorsum of foot**
  Os intercuneiforme
  Os talonaviculare dorsale
  Os calcaneus secondarius
  Os intermetatarsal I
- **Posterior part of foot**
  Os trigonum
- **Lateral part of foot**
  Os calcaneus secondarius
  Os vesalianum pedis
- **Medial part of foot**
  Os tibiale externum (Os naviculare accessorium)
  Os sustentaculi
- **Plantar aspect (sole) of foot**
  Pars peronea metatarsalis I
  Os cuboides secondarius

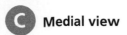

C Medial view

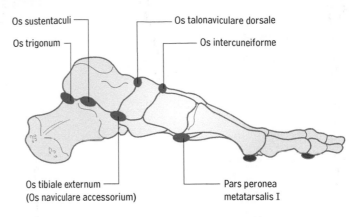

Os sustentaculi
Os trigonum
Os talonaviculare dorsale
Os intercuneiforme
Os tibiale externum (Os naviculare accessorium)
Pars peronea metatarsalis I

D Lateral view

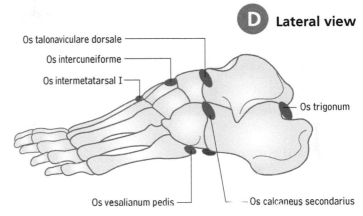

Os talonaviculare dorsale
Os intercuneiforme
Os intermetatarsal I
Os trigonum
Os vesalianum pedis
Os calcaneus secondarius

E

Inferior (plantar) view

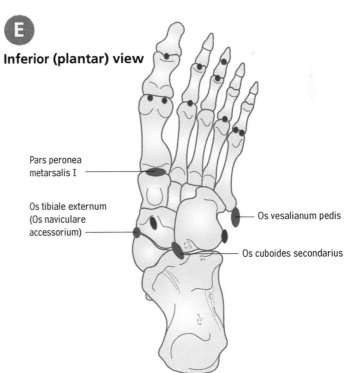

Pars peronea metarsalis I
Os tibiale externum (Os naviculare accessorium)
Os vesalianum pedis
Os cuboides secondarius

C D E Common locations of sesamoid (red) and accessory (blue) bones

Skeleton of the foot *Articulated bones of the left foot*

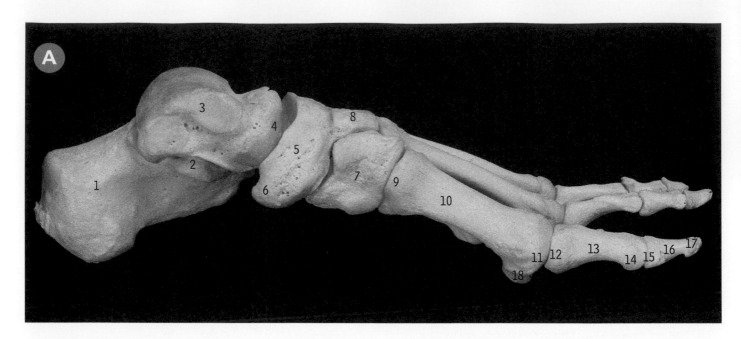

A From the medial side

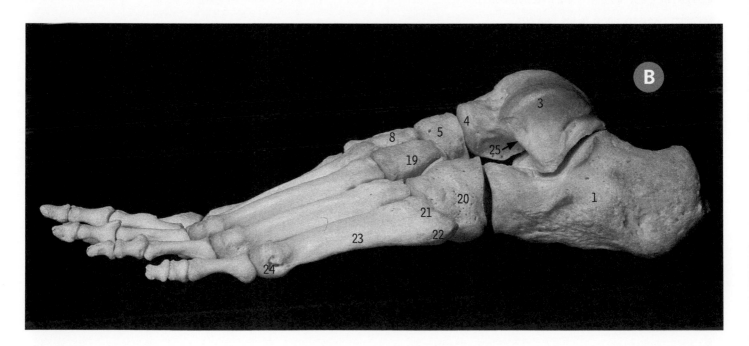

B From the lateral side

1   Body of calcaneus
2   Sustentaculum tali part of calcaneus
3   Body of talus ⎫
4   Head of talus ⎬ of talus
5   Navicular
6   Tuberosity of navicular
7   Medial cuneiform
8   Intermediate cuneiform
9   Base ⎫
10 Body ⎬ of first metatarsal
11 Head ⎭
12 Base ⎫
13 Body ⎬ of proximal phalanx of great toe
14 Head ⎭
15 Base ⎫
16 Body ⎬ of distal phalanx of great toe
17 Head ⎭
18 Sesamoid bone
19 Lateral cuneiform
20 Cuboid
21 Base ⎫
22 Tuberosity ⎬ of fifth metatarsal
23 Body ⎪
24 Head ⎭
25 Tarsal sinus

- When standing (as can be seen from the imprint of a wet foot on the floor or when viewed through a glass plate—see p. 45, **F**) the parts of the foot in contact with the ground are the heel, the lateral margin of the foot, the pads under the metatarsal heads and the pads under the distal part of the toes.
- The medial margin of the foot is not normally in contact with the ground because of the height of the medial longitudinal arch (see pp. 56 and 57). In flat foot the medial arch is lower with an increasingly large imprint on the medial side.
- The body weight when standing is borne by the tuberosity of the calcaneus and the heads of the metatarsals, especially the first (with the sesamoid bones underneath it) and the fifth. As the foot bends forward in walking the other metatarsal heads take increasingly more of the load. With further raising of the heel the toe pads become pressed to the ground and so take some of the weight off the metatarsals.
- Although the forearm and hand have many muscles similar in name and action to those of the leg and foot, their normal use in everyday life is different. In the upper limb the muscles work from above to produce intricate movements of the thumb and fingers in a free limb. In the lower limb the toes must be stabilized on the ground so that muscles can work from below to produce the propulsive movements of walking.

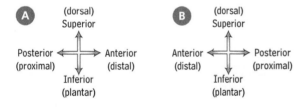

Skeleton of the foot

Bones of the left longitudinal arches, transverse tarsal joint and other joints

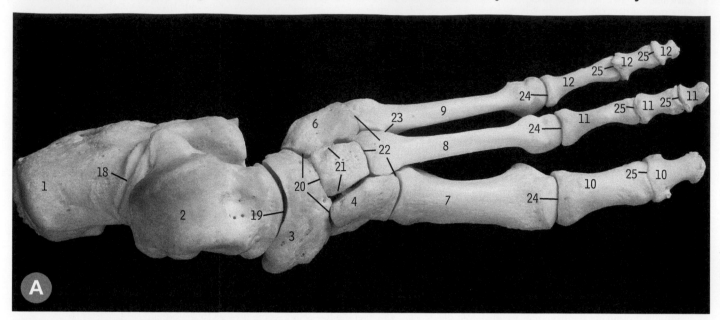

A Bones of the medial longitudinal arch, from above

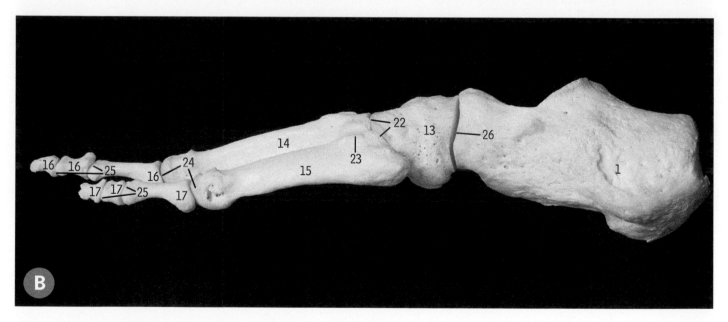

B Bones of the lateral longitudinal arch, from the lateral side

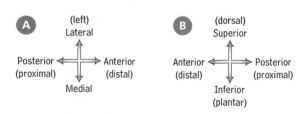

A (left)
Lateral

Posterior ⟵ ⟶ Anterior
(proximal)   (distal)

Medial

B (dorsal)
Superior

Anterior ⟵ ⟶ Posterior
(distal)   (proximal)

Inferior
(plantar)

- The bones of the medial longitudinal arch (**A**) are the calcaneus, talus, navicular, the three cuneiforms and the medial three metatarsal bones.
- The bones of the lateral longitudinal arch (**B**) are the calcaneus, cuboid and the two lateral metatarsal bones.
- The transverse arch is formed by the cuboid and cuneiform bones and the adjacent parts of the five metatarsals (those of each foot forming one half of the whole arch). At the level of the metatarsal heads the arched form is no longer present.
- The medial longitudinal arch is higher than the lateral.
- Although the shape of the individual bones determines the shapes of the arches, the *maintenance* of the arches in the *stationary* foot (standing in the normal upright position) depends largely on the ligaments in the sole (where they are larger and stronger than those on the dorsum). As soon as movement occurs the long tendons and small muscles of the sole assume importance in maintaining the curved forms.
- The many joints of the foot contribute to its function as a *flexible* lever, and the word arch suggests an architectural rigidity that does not exist.
- On the medial side the plantar calcaneonavicular ligament (spring ligament) is of particular importance in supporting the head of the talus, and other structures that help to maintain the medial arch include the plantar aponeurosis, flexor hallucis longus, tibialis anterior and posterior, and the medial parts of flexor digitorum longus and brevis.
- The transverse tarsal joint (midtarsal joint) is the collective name for two joints—the calcaneocuboid joint, and the talonavicular part of the talocalcaneonavicular joint.

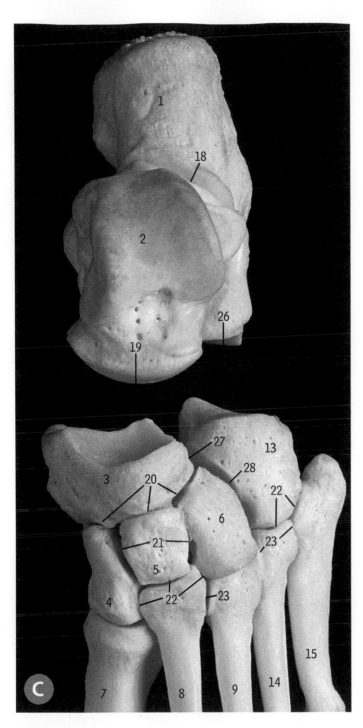

C The transverse tarsal joint, disarticulated, from above

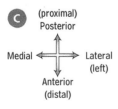

1 Calcaneus
2 Talus
3 Navicular
4 Medial cuneiform
5 Intermediate cuneiform
6 Lateral cuneiform
7 First metatarsal
8 Second metatarsal
9 Third metatarsal
10 Phalanges of great toe
11 Phalanges of second toe
12 Phalanges of third toe
13 Cuboid
14 Fourth metatarsal
15 Fifth metatarsal
16 Phalanges of fourth toe
17 Phalanges of fifth toe
18 Talocalcanean joint
19 Talonavicular part of talocalcaneonavicular joint
20 Cuneonavicular joint
21 Intercuneiform joints
22 Tarsometatarsal joints (cuneometatarsal and cuboideometatarsal)
23 Intermetatarsal joints
24 Metatarsophalangeal joints
25 Interphalangeal joints
26 Calcaneocuboid joint
27 Cuboideonavicular joint
28 Cuneocuboid joint

Foot bones *Left talus*

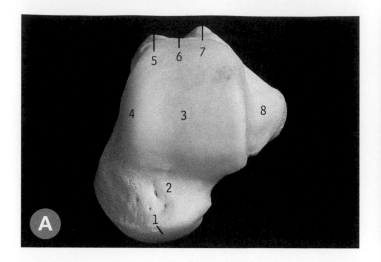

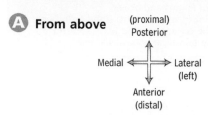

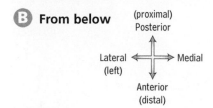

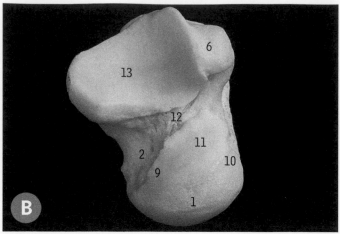

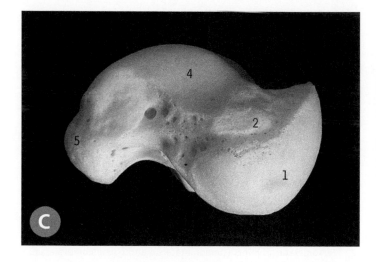

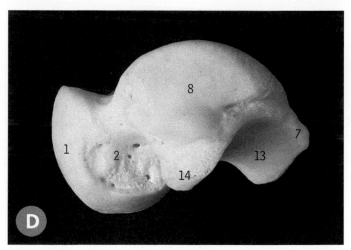

A From above

(proximal)
Posterior

Medial ⟷ Lateral
(left)

Anterior
(distal)

B From below

(proximal)
Posterior

Lateral ⟷ Medial
(left)

Anterior
(distal)

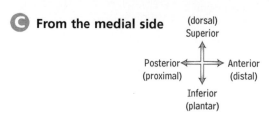

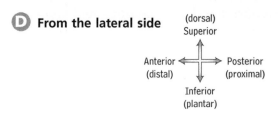

C From the medial side

(dorsal)
Superior

Posterior ⟷ Anterior
(proximal)   (distal)

Inferior
(plantar)

D From the lateral side

(dorsal)
Superior

Anterior ⟷ Posterior
(distal)   (proximal)

Inferior
(plantar)

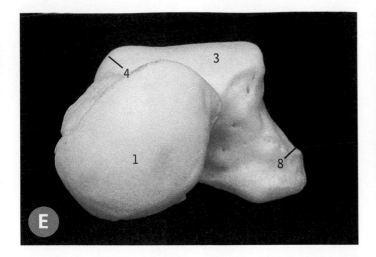

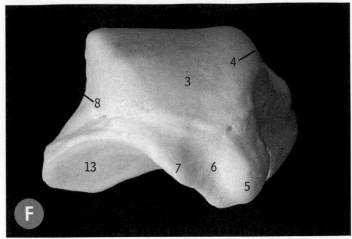

E From the front

(dorsal)
Superior

Medial ⟷ Lateral
(left)

Inferior
(plantar)

F From behind

(dorsal)
Superior

Lateral ⟷ Medial
(left)

Inferior
(plantar)

1 Head with articular surface for navicular
2 Neck
3 Trochlear surface of body, for inferior surface of tibia
4 Surface for medial malleolus
5 Medial tubercle
6 Groove for flexor hallucis longus tendon } of posterior process
7 Lateral tubercle
8 Surface for lateral malleolus
9 Anterior calcanean articular surface
10 Surface for plantar calcaneonavicular (spring) ligament
11 Middle calcanean articular surface
12 Sulcus tali
13 Posterior calcanean articular surface
14 Lateral process

Talus
• The uppermost foot bone, forming the ankle joint with the tibia and fibula.
• Formerly known as the astragalus.
• Articular facets on the upper surface and sides for the tibia and fibula, on the under surface for the calcaneus, and on the anterior surface (head) for the navicular.
• Unique among the foot bones in having no muscles attached to it.

Foot bones *Left talus and the lower ends of the tibia and fibula*

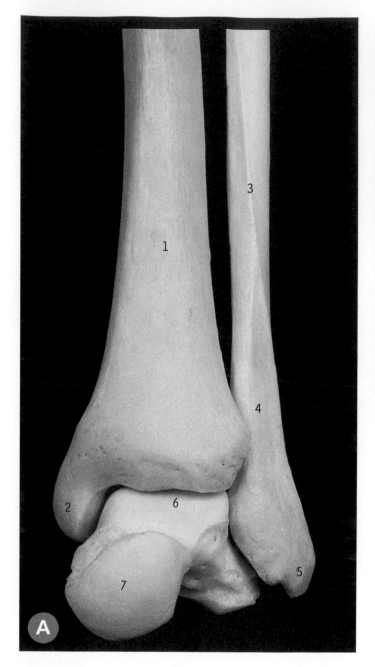

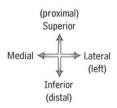

A The talus, tibia and fibula, articulated, from the front

(proximal)
Superior

Medial ←→ Lateral
(left)

Inferior
(distal)

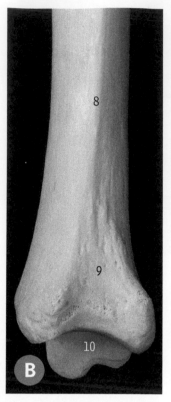

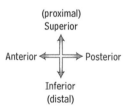

B The tibia from the lateral side

(proximal)
Superior

Anterior ←→ Posterior

Inferior
(distal)

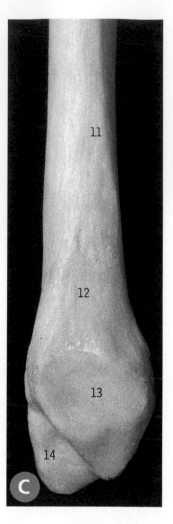

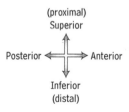

C The fibula from the medial side

(proximal)
Superior

Posterior ←→ Anterior

Inferior
(distal)

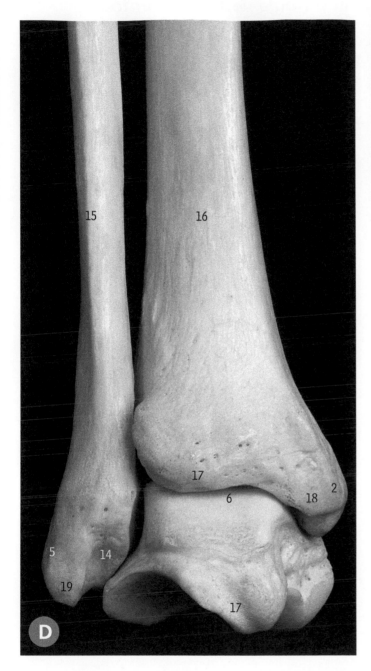

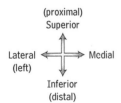

D The talus, tibia and fibula, articulated, from behind

(proximal)
Superior

Lateral ←→ Medial
(left)

Inferior
(distal)

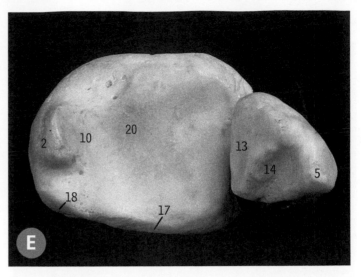

E The tibia and fibula, articulated, from below

Anterior

Medial ←→ Lateral
(left)

Posterior

1 Anterior surface ⎤ of tibia
2 Medial malleolus ⎦
3 Anterior border ⎤
4 Triangular subcutaneous area ⎬ of fibula
5 Lateral malleolus ⎦
6 Trochlear surface of body ⎤ of talus
7 Head ⎦
8 Interosseous border ⎤
9 Fibular notch ⎬ of tibia
10 Articular (lateral) surface of medial malleolus ⎦
11 Interosseous border ⎤
12 Surface for interosseous tibiofibularis ligament ⎥
13 Articular (medial) surface of lateral malleolus ⎬ of fibula
14 Malleolar fossa ⎥
15 Posterior border ⎦
16 Posterior surface of tibia
17 Groove for flexor hallucis longus tendon
18 Groove for tibialis posterior tendon
19 Groove for fibularis (peroneus) brevis tendon
20 Inferior surface of tibia

Foot bones

Left talus and the lower ends of the tibia and fibula, with ligamentous attachments in the ankle region

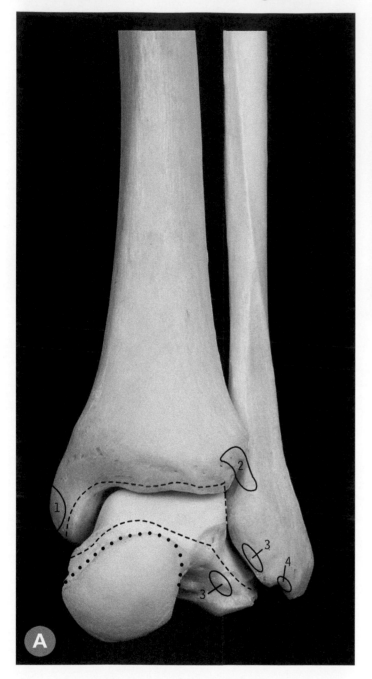

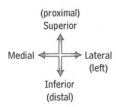

A The talus, tibia and fibula, articulated, from the front

(proximal)
Superior

Medial ←——→ Lateral
(left)

Inferior
(distal)

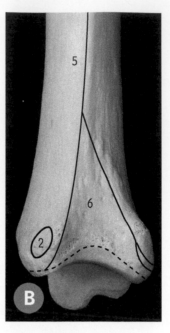

B The tibia from the lateral side

B (proximal)
Superior

Anterior ←——→ Posterior

Inferior
(distal)

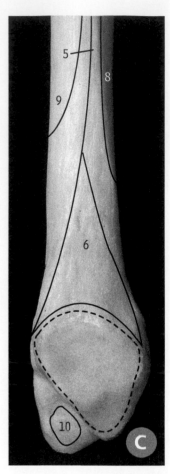

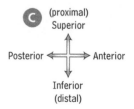

C The fibula from the medial side

C (proximal)
Superior

Posterior ←——→ Anterior

Inferior
(distal)

The attachment of the capsule of the ankle joint is indicated by the dashed line, and that of the talocalcaneonavicular joint is indicated by the dotted line.

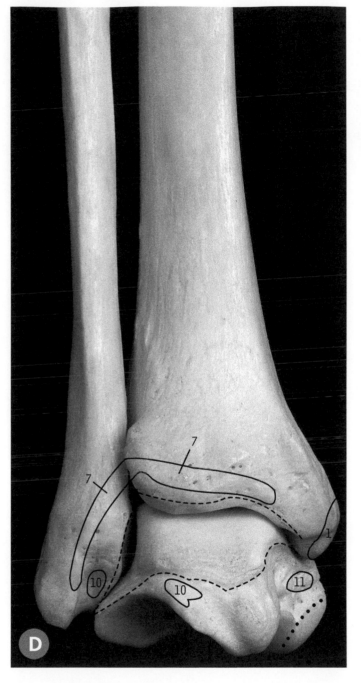

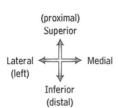

D The talus, tibia and fibula, articulated, from behind

(proximal)
Superior

Lateral ←——→ Medial
(left)

Inferior
(distal)

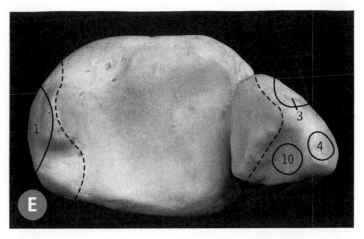

E The tibia and fibula, articulated, from below

Anterior

Medial ←——→ Lateral
(left)

Posterior

1 Medial (deltoid) ligament
2 Anterior tibiofibular ligament
3 Anterior talofibular ligament
4 Calcaneofibular ligament
5 Interosseous membrane
6 Interosseous tibiofibular ligament
7 Posterior tibiofibular ligament
8 Fibularis (*peroneus*) tertius
9 Flexor hallucis longus
10 Posterior talofibular ligament
11 Deep part of medial (deltoid) ligament

- The interosseous tibiofibular ligament (**B** and **C, 6**) is the main bond of union of the inferior tibiofibular joint.

Foot bones

Left talus and the lower ends of the tibia and fibula

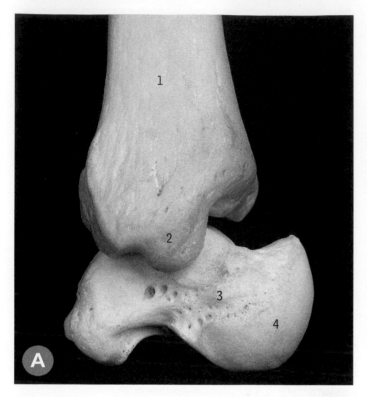

Ⓐ The talus and tibia, articulated, from the medial side

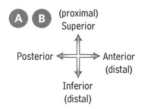

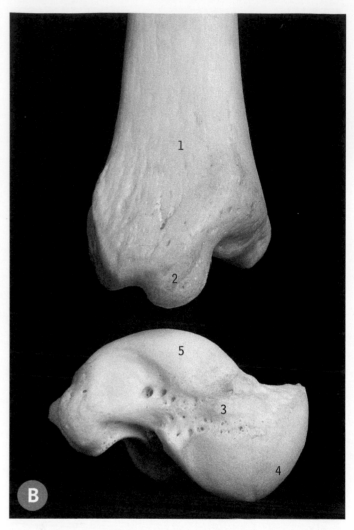

Ⓑ The talus and tibia, disarticulated, from the medial side

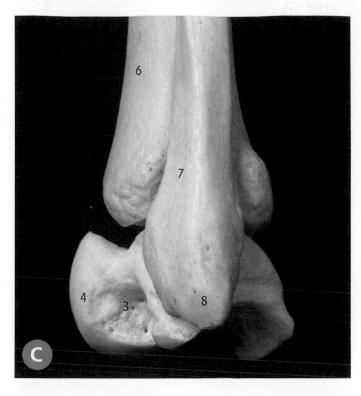

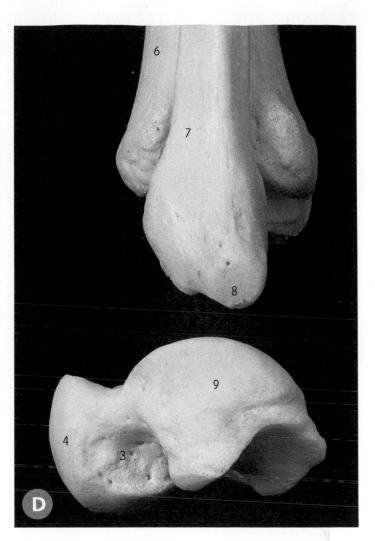

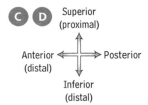

C The talus, tibia and fibula, articulated, from the lateral side

1 Medial surface ⎱ of tibia
2 Medial malleolus ⎰
3 Neck ⎱ of talus
4 Head ⎰
5 Surface for medial malleolus
6 Anterior surface of tibia
7 Triangular subcutaneous surface ⎱ of fibula
8 Lateral malleolus ⎰
9 Surface for lateral malleolus

D The talus disarticulated from the tibia and fibula, from the lateral side

C **D** Superior (proximal)

Anterior (distal) ⟷ Posterior

Inferior (distal)

Foot bones

Left talus and the lower ends of the tibia and fibula, with ligamentous attachments in the ankle region

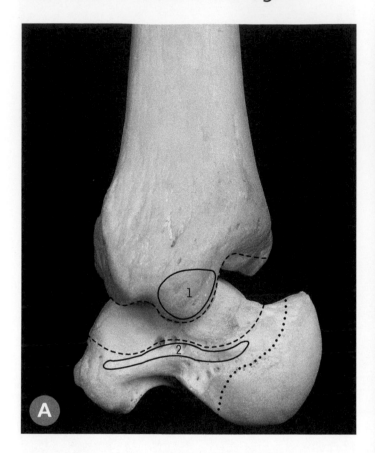

A The talus and tibia, articulated, from the medial side

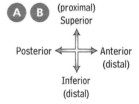

A **B** (proximal)
Superior

Posterior ← → Anterior
(distal)

Inferior
(distal)

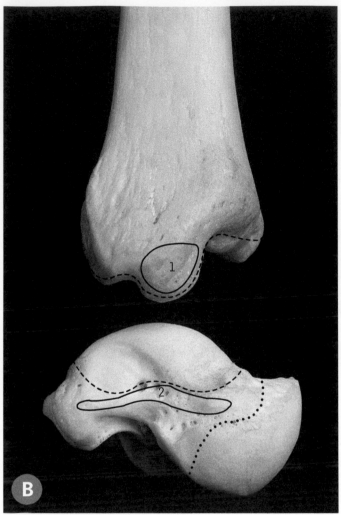

B The talus and tibia, disarticulated, from the medial side

The attachment of the capsule of the ankle joint is indicated by the dashed line, and that of the talocalcaneonavicular joint is indicated by the dotted line.

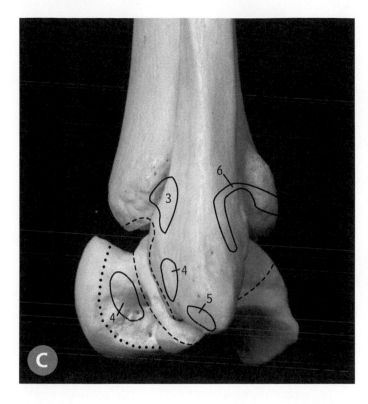

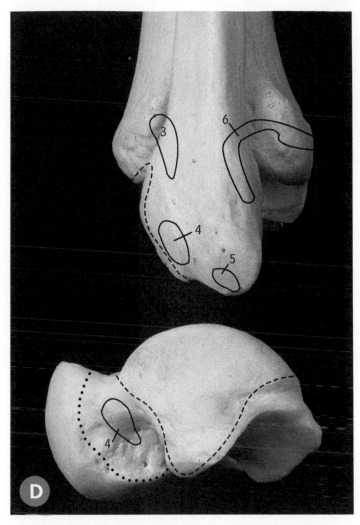

C The talus, tibia and fibula, articulated, from the lateral side

1   Medial (deltoid) ligament
2   Deep part of medial (deltoid) ligament
3   Anterior tibiofibular ligament
4   Anterior talofibular ligament
5   Calcaneofibular ligament
6   Posterior tibiofibular ligament

D The talus disarticulated from the tibia and fibula, from the lateral side by the dotted line.

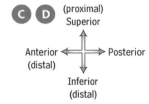

C D (proximal)
Superior

Anterior ←——→ Posterior
(distal)

Inferior
(distal)

Foot bones *Left calcaneus*

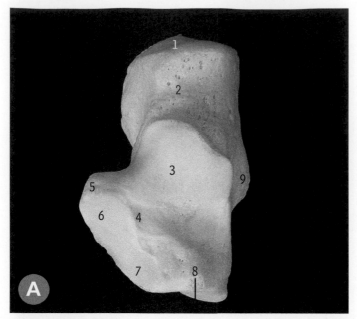

A From above

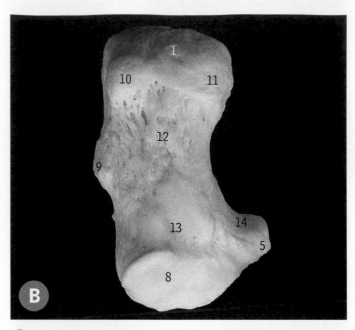

B From below

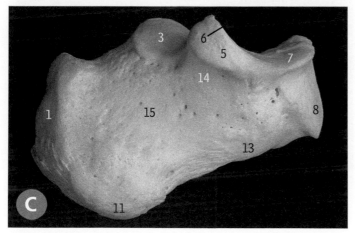

C From the medial side

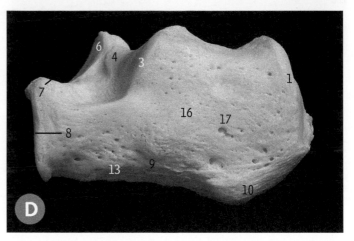

D From the lateral side

1 Posterior surface
2 Dorsal surface
3 Posterior articular surface for talus
4 Sulcus calcanei
5 Sustentaculum tali
6 Middle articular surface for talus ⎱
7 Anterior articular surface for talus ⎰ articular surface for talus
8 Articular surface for cuboid
9 Fibular (*peroneal*) trochlea
10 Lateral process ⎱
11 Medial process ⎰ of tuberosity
12 Plantar surface
13 Anterior tubercle
14 Groove for flexor hallucis longus tendon
15 Medial surface

16 Lateral surface
17 Tubercle for calcaneofibular ligament
18 Surface for bursa
19 Surface for tendo calcaneus
20 Surface for fibrofatty tissue
21 Medial ⎱
22 Lateral ⎰ talocalcanean ligament
23 Tibiocalcanean part of medial (deltoid) ligament
24 Interosseous talocalcanean ligament
25 Inferior extensor retinaculum
26 Cervical ligament
27 Extensor digitorum brevis
28 Calcaneocuboid part
29 Calcaneonavicular part of bifurcate ligament

The capsule of the talocalcanean joint is indicated by the dashed line, and that of the talocalcanean part of the talocalcaneonavicular joint is indicated by the dotted line.

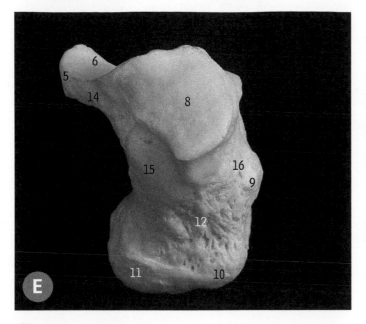

E From the front

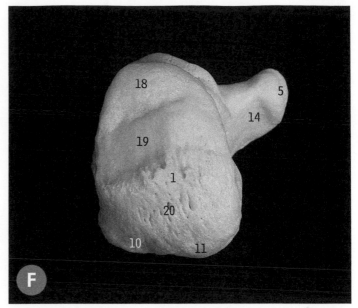

F From behind

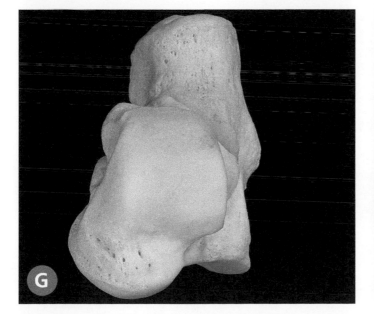

G Articulated with the talus, from above

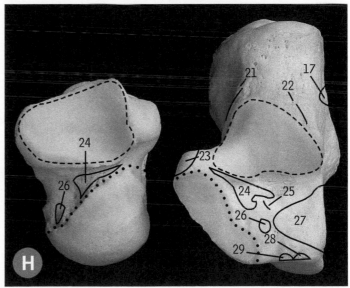

H With the talus disarticulated and turned upside down, with attachments

Calcaneus
- The largest foot bone, forming the heel.
- Formerly known as the calcaneum or os calcis.
- Articular facets on the upper surface for the talus and on the anterior surface for the cuboid.
- Prominent sustentaculum tali projecting medially.
- When the talus and calcaneus are articulated, the sulcus tali (see p. 52, **B12**) and sulcus calcanei (**4**) form the tarsal sinus (sinus tarsi).

Foot bones

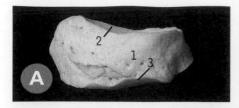

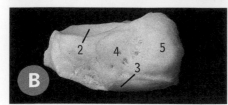

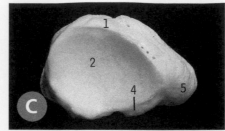

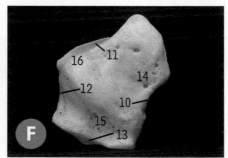

A From above

B From below

C Proximal aspect

D Distal aspect

Left navicular bone

1 Dorsal surface
2 Proximal surface for talus
3 Distal surface for cuneiforms
4 Plantar surface
5 Tuberosity
6 Facet for medial cuneiform
7 Facet for intermediate cuneiform } on distal
8 Facet for lateral cuneiform } surface

> *Navicular bone*
> • Formerly known as the scaphoid bone.
> • Posterior articular facet for the talus; anterior articular facet for the three cuneiforms.

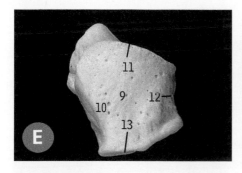

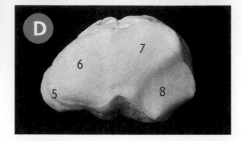

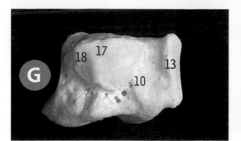

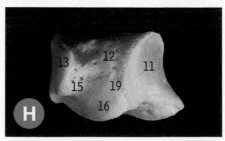

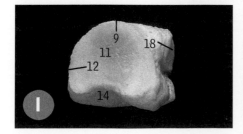

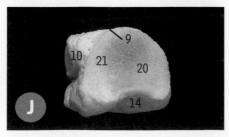

Left cuboid bone

E From above

F From below

G From the medial side

H From the lateral side

I Proximal aspect

J Distal aspect

9 Dorsal surface
10 Medial surface
11 Proximal surface for calcaneus
12 Lateral surface
13 Distal surface
14 Plantar surface
15 Groove for fibularis *(peroneus)* longus tendon
16 Tuberosity
17 Surface for lateral cuneiform
18 Surface for navicular
19 Facet for sesamoid bone in fibularis *(peroneus)* longus tendon
20 Facet for fifth metatarsal } on distal
21 Facet for fourth metatarsal } surface

> *Cuboid bone*
> • Posterior articular facet for the calcaneus; anterior articular facet for the fourth and fifth metatarsals.
> • Groove on the undersurface for the tendon of fibularis (peroneus) longus.

Articulated left cuneiform bones (medial, intermediate and lateral)

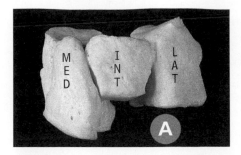

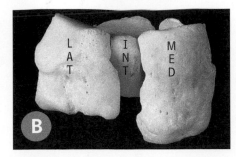

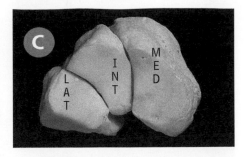

A From above

B From below

C Proximal (navicular) aspect (for distal aspect, see p. 72)

Left medial cuneiform bone

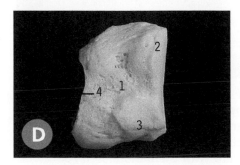

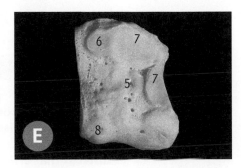

D From the medial side

E From the lateral side

> *Cuneiform bones*
> - Medial (the largest), intermediate (the smallest) and lateral.
> - Situated between the navicular and the first three metatarsals.

1 Medial surface
2 Distal surface for first metatarsal
3 Area for tendon of tibialis anterior
4 Proximal surface for navicular
5 Lateral surface
6 Surface for second metatarsal
7 Surface for intermediate cuneiform
8 Area for fibularis (*peroneus*) longus tendon
9 Medial surface
10 Surface for medial cuneiform
11 Distal surface for second metatarsal
12 Lateral surface
13 Surface for lateral cuneiform
14 Proximal surface for navicular
15 Medial surface
16 Surfaces for second metatarsal
17 Surface for intermediate cuneiform
18 Proximal surface for navicular
19 Lateral surface
20 Surface for cuboid
21 Surface for fourth metatarsal
22 Distal surface for third metatarsal

Left intermediate cuneiform bone

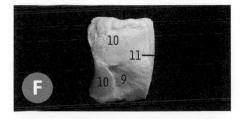

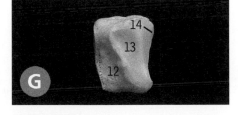

F From the medial side

G From the lateral side

Left lateral cuneiform bone

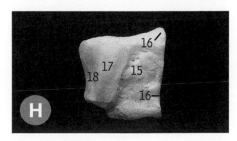

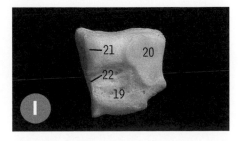

H From the medial side

I From the lateral side

Foot bones

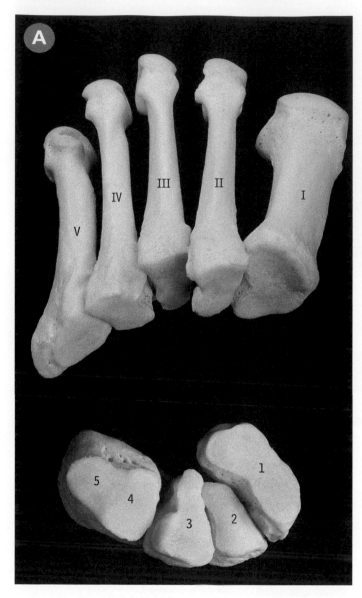

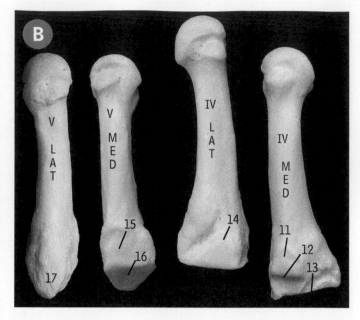

The metatarsal bones are articulated with each other but have been disarticulated from the cuneiform and cuboid bones, which have been rotated to show the surfaces that articulate with the metatarsals. For orientation, see articulated foot (p. 50).

1   Surface of medial cuneiform for first metatarsal
2   Surface of intermediate cuneiform for second metatarsal
3   Surface of lateral cuneiform for third metatarsal
4   Surface of cuboid for fourth metatarsal
5   Surface of cuboid for fifth metatarsal

- The base of the third metatarsal articulates with the lateral cuneiform and the bases of the second and fourth metatarsals.
- The base of the fourth metatarsal articulates with the lateral cuneiform and the cuboid and the base of the fifth metatarsal.
- The base of the fifth metatarsal articulates with the cuboid and the base of the fourth metatarsal.

Ⓐ Left cuneiform, cuboid and metatarsal bones articulated, from above and in front

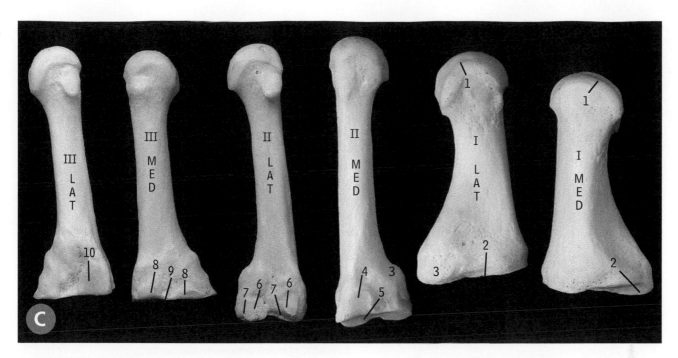

B **C** Left metatarsal bones—numbered I–V with their medial and lateral sides named

The bones are arranged on their sides so that the articular surfaces on the adjacent sides of their bases can be seen; for orientation see articulated foot (p. 50).

1 Groove on head for sesamoid bone
2 Surface for medial cuneiform
3 Area for bursa
4 Surface for medial cuneiform
5 Surface for intermediate cuneiform
6 Surfaces for third metatarsal
7 Surfaces for lateral cuneiform
8 Surfaces for second metatarsal
9 Surface for lateral cuneiform
10 Surface for fourth metatarsal
11 Surface for third metatarsal
12 Surface for lateral cuneiform
13 Surface for cuboid
14 Surface for fifth metatarsal
15 Surface for fourth metatarsal
16 Surface for cuboid
17 Tuberosity of base

Metatarsal bones
- First to fifth, leading to each toe and each with a base (at the proximal or ankle end), body or shaft, and head (at the toe end). Bases of first three articulate with cuneiform bones; bases of fourth and fifth articulate with the cuboid. Heads articulate with bases of proximal phalanges.
- The second, third and fourth metatarsals are longer than the first and fifth; the first is the shortest and the thickest.
- The second metatarsal is the longest bone and its base is recessed between the medial and lateral cuneiforms as well as articulating with the intermediate cuneiform (forming a Keystone). Thus, the second metatarsal is the most rigid of the metatarsals.
- The cuneiforms and bases of the metatarsals are wedge shaped to help form a bony arch.

- Refer to an articulated foot (p. 50) and note the following:
  The base of the first metatarsal articulates with the medial cuneiform. There is normally a bursa but not a joint between the bases of the first and second metatarsals.
  The base of the second metatarsal articulates with all three cuneiforms and with the base of the third metatarsal. This second metatarsal base extends more proximally than the first and third bases—an interlocking device that prevents side-to-side movement.

Lower leg and foot

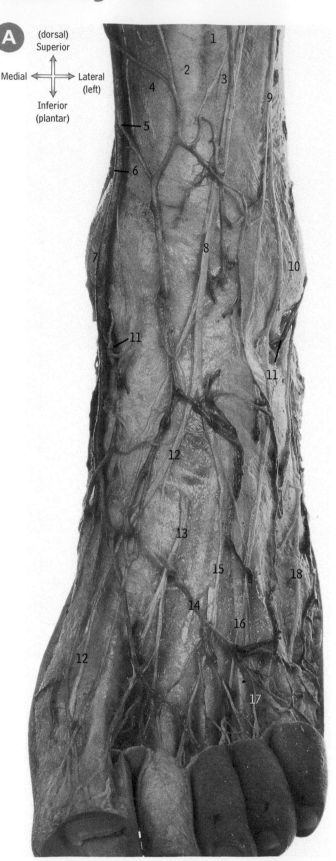

A

(dorsal)
Superior

Medial ⟷ Lateral
(left)

Inferior
(plantar)

A **Superficial vessels and nerves of the left lower leg and foot, from the front**

Skin and superficial connective tissue have been removed to show the superficial vessels and nerves lying on the deep fascia (1). In A the medial side of the dorsal venous arch (14) joins the medial marginal vein of the foot to form the great saphenous vein (5), which runs up in front of the medial malleolus (7). The medial and lateral branches of the superficial fibular *(peroneal)* nerve (8 and 9) pass down on to the dorsum, supplemented on the medial side by the saphenous nerve (6) and on the lateral side by the sural nerve (18). The end of the deep fibular *(peroneal)* nerve (13) perforates the deep fascia to run to the first toe cleft.

1 Deep fascia
2 Tendon of tibialis anterior (under fascia)
3 Tendon of extensor digitorum longus (under fascia)
4 Medial surface of tibia (under fascia)
5 Great saphenous vein
6 Saphenous nerve
7 Medial malleolus
8 Medial branch ⎱ of superficial fibular *(peroneal)* nerve
9 Lateral branch ⎰
10 Lateral malleolus
11 A perforating vein
12 Proper dorsal digital nerve of great toe
13 Medial terminal branch of deep fibular *(peroneal)* nerve
14 Dorsal venous arch
15 Dorsal digital nerve to second cleft
16 Dorsal digital nerve to third cleft
17 Dorsal digital nerve to fourth cleft
18 Sural nerve

- The skin of the first toe cleft is supplied by the *deep* fibular *(peroneal)* nerve (**A13**); the skin of the other clefts is supplied by the *superficial* fibular *(peroneal)* nerve (**A8** and 9).
- The skin behind the ankle and at the back of the heel is supplied on the medial side by the saphenous nerve (**A6**, from the femoral nerve) and the medial calcanean branches (**B8**) of the tibial nerve, and on the lateral side by the sural nerve (**B2**, also from the tibial nerve).
- The saphenous nerve (**A6**) on the medial side of the foot supplies skin as far forward as the metatarsophalangeal joint of the great toe.
- The sural nerve (**A18**) on the lateral side of the foot supplies skin as far forward as the side of the fifth toe.
- The skin of the medial side of the dorsum of the foot, including the region of the medial malleolus, is part of the fourth lumbar dermatome (**Fig. 9**, p. 153). The fifth lumbar dermatome includes the rest of the dorsum, and the first sacral dermatome includes the lateral side of the foot and the lateral malleolar region.
- The *great* saphenous vein (**A5**) passes upward in front of the *medial* malleolus (**A7**).
- The *small* saphenous vein (**B3**) passes upward behind the *lateral* malleolus (**B11**).

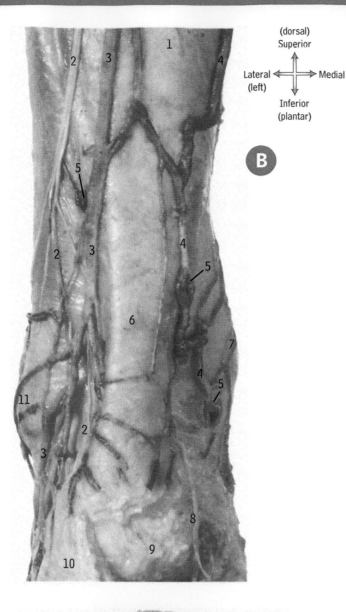

(dorsal)
Superior

Lateral (left) ← → Medial

Inferior (plantar)

B

B Superficial vessels and nerves of the left lower leg and foot, from behind

In B the most obvious structure is the tendo calcaneus (Achilles tendon, 6), running down to be attached to the back of the calcaneus (9). The small saphenous vein (3) and sural nerve (2) with their tributaries and branches are behind the lateral malleolus (11). On both sides but especially the medial, there are some typical perforating veins (5), piercing the deep fascia to form communications between the superficial and deep veins. The posterior arch vein (4) unites several of the perforators on the medial side.

1 Deep fascia
2 Sural nerve
3 Small saphenous vein
4 Posterior arch vein
5 A perforating vein
6 Tendo calcaneus (under fascia)
7 Medial malleolus
8 Medial calcanean nerve
9 Posterior surface of calcaneus
10 Fibrofatty tissue of heel
11 Lateral malleolus

C Axial cross section of the left leg above the level of the upper part of B

The section in C is viewed from below, looking from the ankle toward the knee. Tibialis posterior (13) is the deepest of the calf muscles (immediately behind the interosseous membrane, (5) with the tibial nerve (19) behind it and the posterior tibial vessels (20) more medially, between flexor digitorum longus (21) and soleus (14). The fibular (*peroneal*) artery (12) is adjacent to flexor hallucis longus (11) behind the fibula (8). Note the (unlabeled) dilated veins within and deep to soleus (14); they are the site for potentially dangerous deep venous thrombosis. In the anterior compartment, in front of the interosseous membrane (5), the anterior tibial vessels (3) and deep fibular (*peroneal*) nerve (4) are between tibialis anterior (2) and extensor hallucis longus (6).

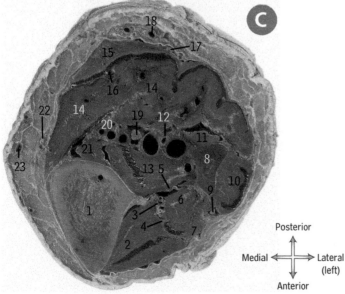

C

Posterior

Medial ← → Lateral (left)

Anterior

1 Tibia	11 Flexor hallucis longus
2 Tibialis anterior	12 Fibular (*peroneal*) artery
3 Anterior tibial vessels	13 Tibialis posterior
4 Deep fibular (*peroneal*) nerve	14 Soleus
5 Interosseous membrane	15 Gastrocnemius
6 Extensor hallucis longus	16 Plantaris tendon
7 Extensor digitorum longus	17 Sural nerve
8 Fibula	18 Small saphenous vein
9 Superficial fibular (*peroneal*) nerve	19 Tibial nerve
10 Fibularis (*peroneus*) longus and brevis	20 Posterior tibial vessels
	21 Flexor digitorum longus
	22 Saphenous nerve
	23 Great saphenous vein

Lower leg and foot

This medial view emphasizes the position of the great saphenous vein (3) in front of the medial malleolus (5), with branches of the saphenous nerve (4) lying both in front of and behind the vein. There are perforating veins (9) behind the malleolus and joining the posterior arch vein (12) and a large medial calcanean branch (10) of the tibial nerve running down to the skin of the heel.

- In the specimen shown on pp. 74–77 some of the superficial veins are rather dilated and tortuous, but this has served to emphasize the posterior arch vein and perforating veins.
- The perforating veins (**A9, B8**) serve as communications between the superficial veins (above the deep fascia) and deep veins (below the fascia). Many of these communicating vessels possess valves that direct the flow of blood from superficial to deep; venous return from the limb is then brought about by the pumping action of the muscles (which are all below the deep fascia). If the valves become incompetent or the deep veins are blocked, pressure in the superficial veins increases and they become varicose (from the Latin for an enlarged and tortuous vessel).
- Perforating veins are variable in number and position but the most constant in the lower leg (**A9**) are near the posterior border of the tibia, one just below and one just above the medial malleolus (**A5**). The posterior arch vein (**A12**) unites these and perhaps other perforators and drains usually into the great saphenous vein below the knee.

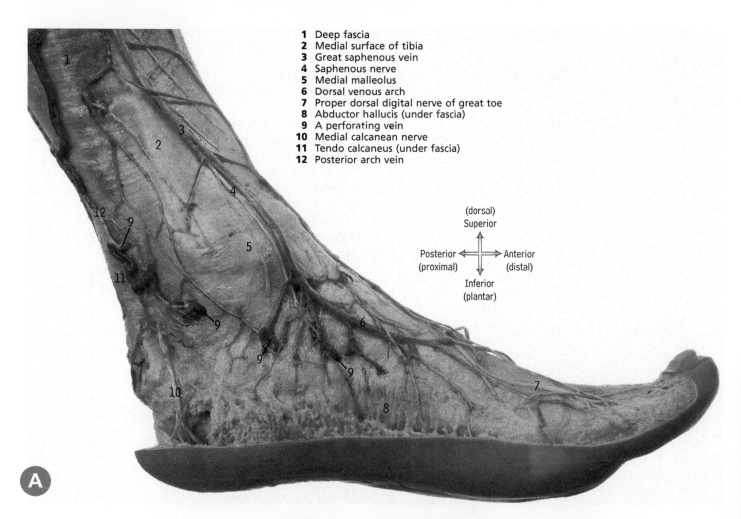

1 Deep fascia
2 Medial surface of tibia
3 Great saphenous vein
4 Saphenous nerve
5 Medial malleolus
6 Dorsal venous arch
7 Proper dorsal digital nerve of great toe
8 Abductor hallucis (under fascia)
9 A perforating vein
10 Medial calcanean nerve
11 Tendo calcaneus (under fascia)
12 Posterior arch vein

(dorsal)
Superior

Posterior ⟷ Anterior
(proximal)   (distal)

Inferior
(plantar)

A Superficial vessels and nerves of the left lower leg and foot, from the medial side

The medial and lateral branches of the superficial fibular *(peroneal)* nerve (1 and 2) run on to the dorsum of the foot. Behind the lateral malleolus (7) are the small saphenous vein (5) and sural nerve (4). The tendon of fibularis *(peroneus)* longus (3) shines through the deep fascia above the malleolus.

- The superficial veins of the dorsum include dorsal digital and dorsal metatarsal veins, which join a dorsal venous arch (**B12**). The ends of the arch join medial and lateral marginal veins that run upward to become the great and small saphenous veins, respectively. (In **A** there is no obvious medial marginal vein, but there is a lateral marginal vein in **B10**.)
- The deep veins run with the deep arteries. The larger arteries in the leg are usually accompanied by a pair of veins (venae comitantes).
- Lymph vessels, resembling narrow, thin-walled veins, accompany many arteries and veins, both superficial and deep. There are no lymph nodes in the foot; most of the lymphatic drainage of the lower limb is to inguinal nodes, but some lymphatic vessels drain into six or seven nodes that lie in the fat of the popliteal fossa. (Occasionally there is a single node beside the upper end of the anterior tibial artery in front of the interosseous membrane.)
- For details of the lymphatic system of the lower Limb see pp. 163–167.

1 Medial branch ⎫ of superficial fibular *(peroneal)* nerve
2 Lateral branch ⎭
3 Deep fascia over fibularis (peroneus) longus tendon
4 Sural nerve
5 Small saphenous vein
6 Tendo calcaneus (under fascia)
7 Lateral malleolus
8 A perforating vein
9 Extensor digitorum brevis (under fascia)
10 Lateral marginal vein
11 Abductor digiti minimi (under fascia)
12 Dorsal venous arch

(dorsal)
Superior

Anterior ←→ Posterior
(distal)   (proximal)

Inferior
(plantar)

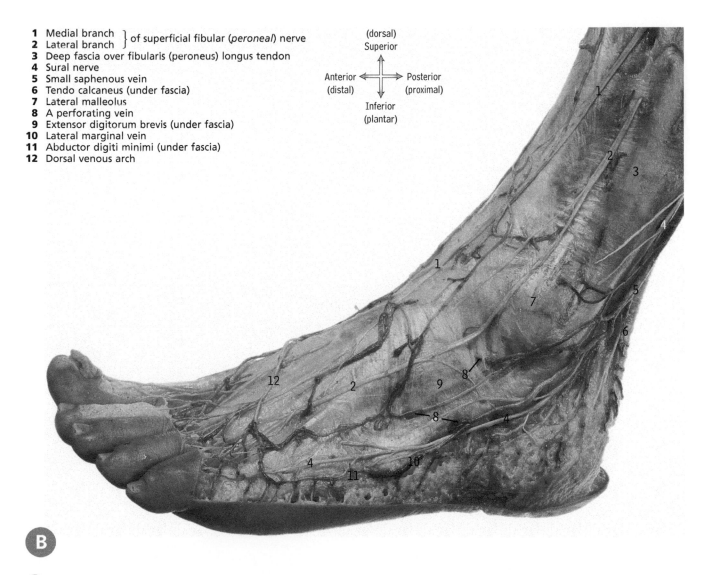

B

B Superficial vessels and nerves of the left lower leg and foot, from the lateral side

Deep fascia of the foot

Deep fascia of the right lower leg and foot, from the front and the right

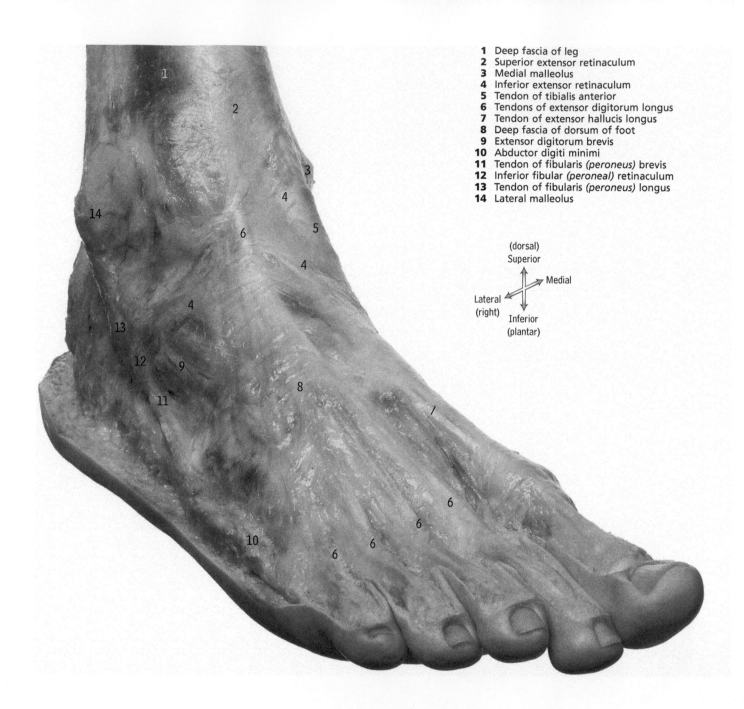

1 Deep fascia of leg
2 Superior extensor retinaculum
3 Medial malleolus
4 Inferior extensor retinaculum
5 Tendon of tibialis anterior
6 Tendons of extensor digitorum longus
7 Tendon of extensor hallucis longus
8 Deep fascia of dorsum of foot
9 Extensor digitorum brevis
10 Abductor digiti minimi
11 Tendon of fibularis (peroneus) brevis
12 Inferior fibular (peroneal) retinaculum
13 Tendon of fibularis (peroneus) longus
14 Lateral malleolus

(dorsal)
Superior

Medial

Lateral
(right)

Inferior
(plantar)

All superficial tissues, including vessels and nerves, have been removed to display the deep fascia. It is thickened in places to form the retinacula (2, 4—see notes), which keep tendons in their proper places; compare with the dissections on pp. 80–83 in which the fascia has been removed to leave only the retinacula. Here, with all the deep fascia intact, tendons and muscles can be seen shining through it.

- The retinacula of the ankle and foot are localized thickenings of deep fascia, which keep tendons in place.
- There are two extensor retinacula (superior and inferior), a flexor retinaculum and two fibular (*peroneal*) retinacula (superior and inferior).
- The superior extensor retinaculum (2) is a band about 4 cm broad and is attached to the lower ends of the anterior borders of the tibia and fibula (see pp. 80, **A7** and 76, **A12**).
- The inferior extensor retinaculum (4) is shaped like a letter Y lying on its side (see pp. 80, **A9**; 82, **A15**; and 83, **B13**).

  The common stem of the Y is on the lateral side and is attached to the upper surface of the calcaneus in front of the sulcus calcanei. The tendons of extensor digitorum longus and fibularis (*peroneus*) tertius (with a common synovial sheath) pass beneath it.

  The upper band of the Y continues upward and medially from the common stem over the deep fibular (*peroneal*) nerve and anterior tibial vessels, then forms a loop to enclose the extensor hallucis longus tendon (within a synovial sheath), finally becoming attached to the medial malleolus after passing either superficial or deep to the tendon of tibialis anterior (within a synovial sheath).

  The lower band of the Y continues downward and medially from the common stem, passing over the terminal branches of the deep fibular (*peroneal*) nerve, the dorsalis pedis vessels and the tendons of extensor hallucis longus (within a synovial sheath) and tibialis anterior, to blend with the plantar aponeurosis overlying abductor hallucis.

- For the flexor retinaculum, see p. 82.
- For the fibular (*peroneal*) retinacula, see p. 83.

Dorsum and back of the foot

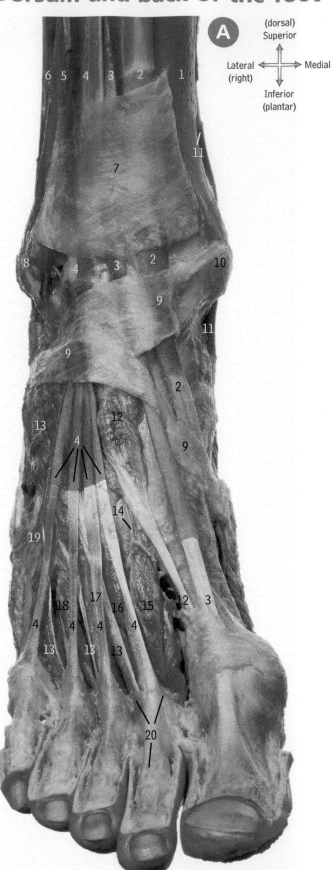

(dorsal)
Superior

Lateral (right) ←→ Medial

Inferior (plantar)

A Superficial dissection of the right lower leg and dorsum of the foot, from the front

Most of the deep fascia has been removed, leaving only the retinacula (7 and 9). The most prominent structures are the long tendons of the extensor muscles (2, 3 and 4) running down from the leg; the synovial sheaths surrounding the tendons in this specimen (which is also shown on pp. 82 and 83) have been emphasized by blue tissue. Extensor digitorum brevis (13, with extensor hallucis brevis, 12—see notes) is the only muscle to arise on the dorsum of the foot.

- Extensor digitorum longus (4) has four tendons that pass to the second, third, fourth and fifth toes.
- Extensor digitorum brevis (13) has four tendons that pass to the great, second, third and fourth toes. The part of the muscle that serves the great toe is known as extensor hallucis brevis (12).
- The dorsal digital expansions (extensor expansions, 20) are derived from the tendons of extensor digitorum longus (4) as they pass over the metatarsophalangeal joints onto the dorsum of the proximal phalanges. They are each triangular in shape with the apex directed distally.
  On the second, third and fourth toes the basal angles of the expansions receive tendons from two interossei and one lumbrical muscle, and the central part of the base receives a tendon of extensor digitorum brevis (13). On the fifth toe one interosseus and one lumbrical tendon are attached.
  The central part of the apex is inserted into the base of the middle phalanx, while two collateral parts run farther forward to be inserted into the base of the distal phalanx (see p. 52, **A16** and 17).
- The order of the structures that pass beneath the superior extensor retinaculum and in front of the ankle joint from the medial to the lateral side is:
  Tibialis anterior tendon (with a synovial sheath) (2)
  Extensor hallucis longus tendon (with no synovial sheath) (3)
  Anterior tibial artery and venae comitantes ⎤ Hidden between
  Deep fibular (peroneal) nerve ⎦ 3 and 4
  Extensor digitorum longus tendon (with no synovial sheath) (4)
  Fibularis (peroneus) tertius tendon (with no synovial sheath) (hidden by 4)

1 Medial surface of tibia	**10** Medial malleolus
2 Tibialis anterior	**11** Tibialis posterior
3 Extensor hallucis longus	**12** Extensor hallucis brevis
4 Extensor digitorum longus	**13** Extensor digitorum brevis
5 Subcutaneous surface of fibula	**14** Dorsalis pedis artery
6 Fibularis (peroneus) brevis	**15** First dorsal interosseus
7 Superior extensor retinaculum	**16** Second dorsal interosseus
8 Lateral malleolus	**17** Third dorsal interosseus
9 Inferior extensor retinaculum	**18** Fourth dorsal interosseus
	19 Fibularis (peroneus) tertius
	20 Dorsal digital expansion

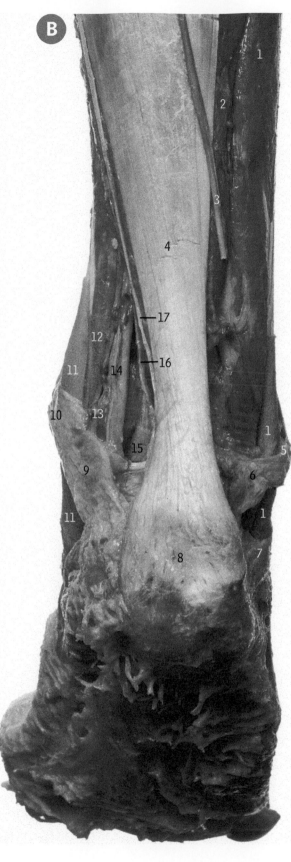

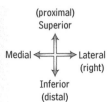

(proximal)
Superior

Medial ←——→ Lateral
(right)

Inferior
(distal)

B Superficial dissection of the back of the right lower leg and foot

C Palpation of the dorsalis pedis pulse. The dorsalis pedis pulse can be felt on a line from midway between the malleoli (5 and 10) toward the first toe cleft

D Palpation of the posterior tibial pulse. The posterior tibial pulse can be felt behind the medial malleolus (10) and 2.5 cm in front of the Achilles tendon (4)

The deep fascia has been removed, leaving only the flexor and fibular (*peroneal*) retinacula (6, 7 and 9). The Achilles tendon (4) passes down to the back of the calcaneus (8). Flexor tendons (11, 12 and 15) lie behind the medial malleolus (10) and fibular (*peroneal*) tendons (1) behind the lateral malleolus (5).

1 Fibularis (peroneus) longus overlapping fibularis (peroneus) brevis
2 Soleus
3 Sural nerve
4 Tendo calcaneus (Achilles tendon)
5 Lateral malleolus
6 Superior ⎫ fibular (*peroneal*) retinaculum
7 Inferior ⎭
8 Posterior surface of calcaneus
9 Flexor retinaculum
10 Medial malleolus
11 Tibialis posterior
12 Flexor digitorum longus
13 Posterior tibial artery and venae comitantes
14 Tibial nerve
15 Flexor hallucis longus
16 Medial calcanean nerve
17 Plantaris tendon

• For the order of the structures behind the medial malleolus, see the notes on the flexor retinaculum on p. 82.

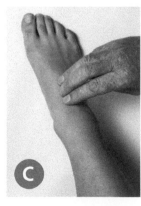

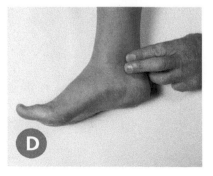

Dorsum and sides of the foot

The synovial sheaths of tendons have been emphasised by blue tissue. The deep fascia has been removed, leaving the flexor retinaculum (12), with part of the inferior extensor retinaculum (15) also visible in this view. The posterior tibial vessels (4) and the tibial nerve (5) lie between the tendons of flexor digitorum longus (3) in front and flexor hallucis longus (6) behind. The prominent muscle on the medial side of the sole is abductor hallucis (14).

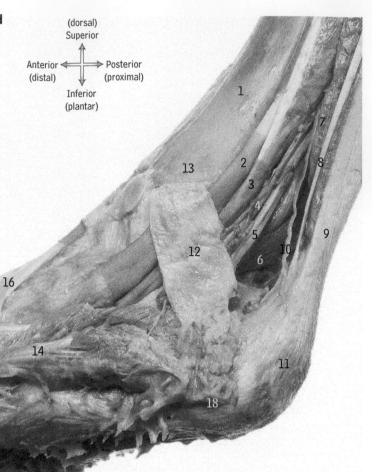

(dorsal)
Superior

Anterior ←——→ Posterior
(distal)   (proximal)

Inferior
(plantar)

A Superficial dissection of the right lower leg and foot, from the medial side

1 Medial surface of tibia
2 Tibialis posterior
3 Flexor digitorum longus
4 Posterior tibial artery and venae comitantes
5 Tibial nerve
6 Flexor hallucis longus
7 Soleus
8 Plantaris tendon
9 Tendo calcaneus
10 Medial calcanean nerve
11 Posterior surface of calcaneus
12 Flexor retinaculum
13 Medial malleolus
14 Abductor hallucis
15 Inferior extensor retinaculum
16 Tibialis anterior
17 Extensor hallucis longus
18 Medial process of tuberosity of calcaneus

- The flexor retinaculum (**12**) passes from the medial malleolus to the medial process of the tuberosity of the calcaneus (**18**).
  Deep to the retinaculum are four connective tissue compartments—three for tendons and one for neurovascular structures. The order of the structures behind the medial malleolus from before backwards is:

  Tibialis posterior tendon (**2**, within a synovial sheath)
  Flexor digitorum longus tendon (**3**, within a synovial sheath)
  Posterior tibial artery and venae comitantes (**4**)
  Tibial nerve (**5**)
  Flexor hallucis longus tendon (**6**, within a synovial sheath).

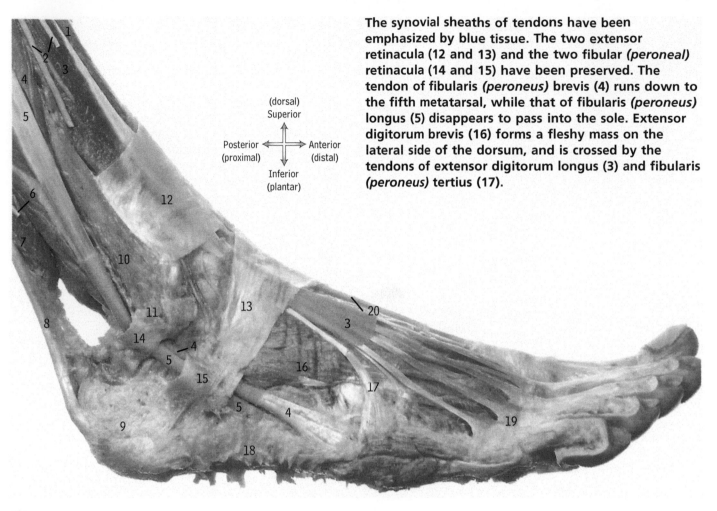

The synovial sheaths of tendons have been emphasized by blue tissue. The two extensor retinacula (12 and 13) and the two fibular *(peroneal)* retinacula (14 and 15) have been preserved. The tendon of fibularis *(peroneus)* brevis (4) runs down to the fifth metatarsal, while that of fibularis *(peroneus)* longus (5) disappears to pass into the sole. Extensor digitorum brevis (16) forms a fleshy mass on the lateral side of the dorsum, and is crossed by the tendons of extensor digitorum longus (3) and fibularis *(peroneus)* tertius (17).

(dorsal)
Superior

Posterior ⟵⟶ Anterior
(proximal)   (distal)

Inferior
(plantar)

B **Superficial dissection of the right lower leg and foot, from the lateral side**

1 Tibialis anterior
2 Medial and lateral branches of superficial fibular (peroneal) nerve
3 Extensor digitorum longus
4 Fibularis (peroneus) brevis
5 Fibularis (peroneus) longus
6 Sural nerve
7 Soleus
8 Tendo calcaneus
9 Lateral surface of calcaneus
10 Subcutaneous area of fibula
11 Lateral malleolus
12 Superior } extensor retinaculum
13 Inferior
14 Superior } fibular (peroneal) retinaculum
15 Inferior
16 Extensor digitorum brevis
17 Fibularis (peroneus) tertius
18 Abductor digiti minimi
19 A dorsal digital expansion
20 Extensor hallucis longus

- The superior fibular *(peroneal)* retinaculum (14) passes from the lateral malleolus (11) to the lateral surface of the calcaneus (9). Deep to the retinaculum are the tendons of fibularis *(peroneus)* brevis (4) and fibularis *(peroneus)* longus (5) (both within a single synovial sheath). The brevis tendon is in front of the longus tendon.
- The inferior fibular *(peroneal)* retinaculum (15) continues backwards and downwards from the common stem of the inferior extensor retinaculum (13) to the lateral surface of the calcaneus (9), with an intermediate attachment to the fibular *(peroneal)* trochlea (see p. 68, **B9**).
   Deep to the retinaculum above and in front of the trochlea is the fibularis *(peroneus)* brevis tendon (4, within its own synovial sheath), while below and behind the trochlea is the fibularis *(peroneus)* longus tendon (5, within its own synovial sheath).

Dorsum and sides of the foot

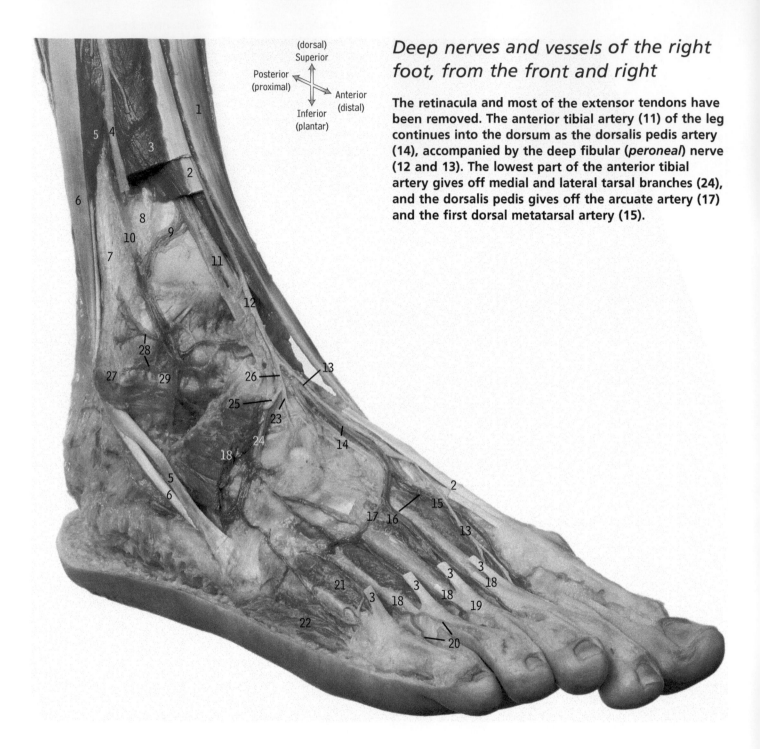

(dorsal) Superior

Posterior (proximal)

Anterior (distal)

Inferior (plantar)

Deep nerves and vessels of the right foot, from the front and right

The retinacula and most of the extensor tendons have been removed. The anterior tibial artery (11) of the leg continues into the dorsum as the dorsalis pedis artery (14), accompanied by the deep fibular (*peroneal*) nerve (12 and 13). The lowest part of the anterior tibial artery gives off medial and lateral tarsal branches (24), and the dorsalis pedis gives off the arcuate artery (17) and the first dorsal metatarsal artery (15).

1 Tibialis anterior
2 Extensor hallucis longus
3 Extensor digitorum longus
4 Lateral branch of superficial fibular (peroneal) nerve
5 Fibularis (peroneus) brevis
6 Fibularis (peroneus) longus
7 Subcutaneous surface of fibula
8 Interosseous membrane
9 Lateral malleolar artery and venae comitantes
10 Perforating branch of fibular (peroneal) artery
11 Anterior tibial artery
12 Deep fibular (peroneal) nerve
13 Medial terminal branch of 12
14 Dorsalis pedis artery
15 First dorsal metatarsal artery

16 Deep plantar artery
17 Arcuate artery
18 Extensor digitorum brevis (hallucis brevis to great toe)
19 Dorsal digital expansion
20 Dorsal digital artery
21 Fourth dorsal interosseus
22 Abductor digiti minimi
23 Interosseous branch of 26
24 Lateral tarsal vessels
25 Nerve to extensor digitorum brevis
26 Lateral terminal branch of 12
27 Lateral malleolus
28 Lateral malleolar arterial rete
29 Anterior talofibular ligament

- As the anterior tibial artery (11) crosses the lower margin of the tibia at the ankle joint it becomes the dorsalis pedis artery (14).
- After giving off medial and lateral tarsal branches (24) the dorsalis pedis artery (14) ends by dividing into the first dorsal metatarsal and the arcuate arteries (15 and 17).
- The first dorsal metatarsal artery (15) gives off a deep plantar (perforating) branch (16) that passes into the sole between the two heads of the first dorsal interosseus muscle to complete the plantar arch with the deep part of the lateral plantar artery (see p. 93, B20).
- The arcuate artery (17) gives off the other three dorsal metatarsal arteries, and all the metatarsal arteries give dorsal digital branches.
- Sometimes the perforating branch of the fibular (peroneal) artery (10), which anastomoses with the lateral tarsal and arcuate arteries (24 and 17), is large and replaces the dorsalis pedis artery, which is absent in about 12% of feet.
- Theoretically each side of each toe has a dorsal digital artery and a plantar digital artery but the individual vessels soon become merged into an anastomotic network.
- For a summary of the branches of the dorsalis pedis artery, see p. 154.

Deep dissection of the dorsum

Joints beneath the talus of the left foot

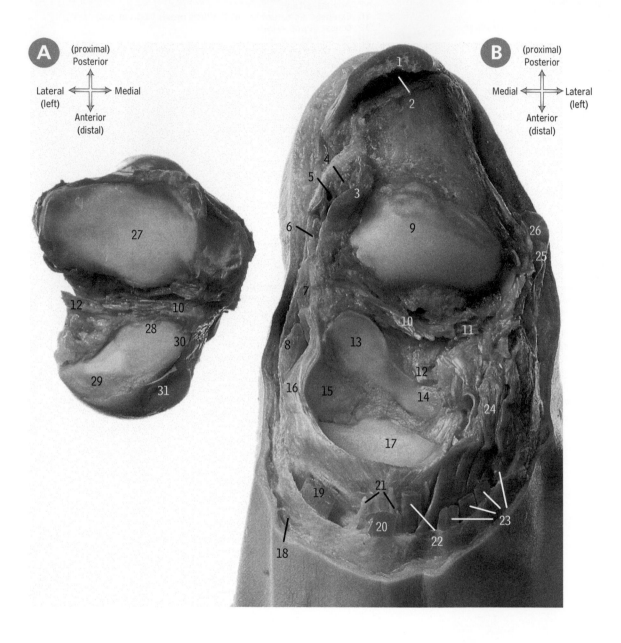

The talus has been removed from the left foot and turned upside down to lie adjacent, so exposing the reciprocal joint surfaces. At the back the concave posterior articular surface of the talus (27) forms the talocalcanean joint with the convex posterior articular surface of the calcaneus (9). At the front are the various parts of the talocalcaneonavicular joint (see notes). The convex middle and anterior surfaces of the talus (28 and 29) articulate with the concave middle and anterior surfaces of the calcaneus (13 and 14), with part of the anterior surface of the talus (30) articulating with cartilage in the upper surface of the spring ligament (15). The convex head of the talus (31) articulates with the concave posterior surface of the navicular bone (17).

1 Tendo calcaneus
2 Bursa
3 Flexor hallucis longus
4 Lateral plantar nerve
5 Posterior tibial vessels
6 Medial plantar nerve
7 Flexor digitorum longus
8 Tibialis posterior
9 Posterior articular surface of calcaneus
10 Interosseous talocalcanean ligament
11 Inferior extensor retinaculum
12 Cervical ligament
13 Middle ⎫ articular surface of calcaneus
14 Anterior ⎭
15 Cartilage in plantar calcaneonavicular (spring) ligament
16 Medial (deltoid) ligament of ankle joint
17 Posterior articular surface of navicular
18 Great saphenous vein
19 Tibialis anterior
20 Extensor hallucis longus
21 Deep fibular (peroneal) nerve
22 Dorsalis pedis artery
23 Extensor digitorum longus
24 Extensor digitorum brevis
25 Fibularis (peroneus) brevis
26 Fibularis (peroneus) longus
27 Posterior ⎫
28 Middle ⎬ calcanean articular surface of talus
29 Anterior ⎭
30 Surface for plantar calcaneonavicular (spring) ligament
31 Surface for navicular

- Apart from the joints of the toes, the most important joints of the rest of the foot are those related to the talus.
- Above the talus is the ankle joint (properly known as the talocrural joint), between the trochlear surface of the talus and the lower ends of the tibia and fibula.
- Below the talus there are two separate joints. Toward the back is the talocalcanean joint (alternatively known as the subtalar joint—but see below), between the posterior articular surfaces of the lower part of the talus (27) and upper part of the calcaneus (9). In front is the talocalcaneonavicular joint, which is a two-part joint between the front of the head of the talus (31) and the navicular (17) (the talonavicular part of this joint), and the articulations of the undersurface of the talus (28–30) with the anterior and middle facets on the upper surface of the calcaneus (14 and 13) and the upper surface of the plantar calcaneonavicular (spring) ligament (15) (the talocalcanean part of this joint).
- Unfortunately there is some confusion of terminology, for clinicians frequently use 'subtalar joint' as a collective name for both joints beneath the talus, not just the posterior one.

Sole of the foot *Plantar aponeurosis of the left foot*

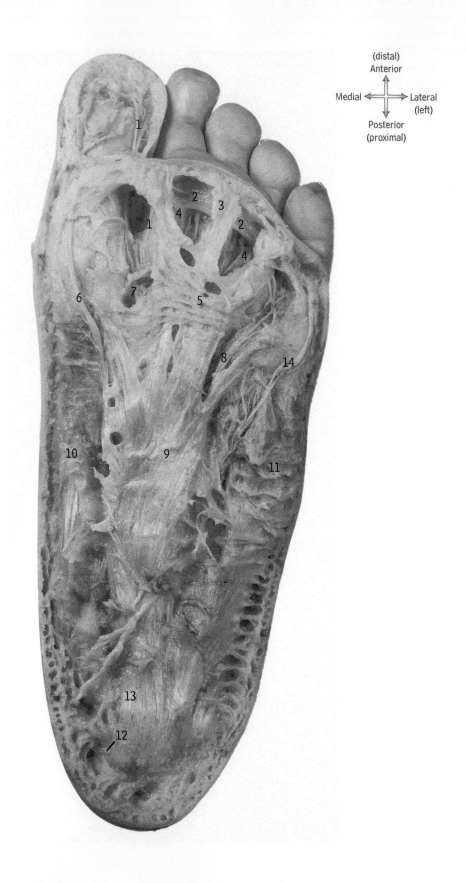

Skin and subcutaneous tissue have been removed to show the thick central part of the plantar aponeurosis (9) and the thinner medial and lateral parts (10 and 11). The numerous strands and septa of fibrous tissue that attach the aponeurosis to the overlying tissues have not been removed to make a tidy dissection; they are an important part of the anatomy of the sole, binding adjacent tissues together.

- **Nerve supplies** in the sole include the following:
  Cutaneous: the medial plantar nerve supplies the medial part of the sole and the medial three and a half toes; the lateral plantar nerve supplies the lateral part of the sole and lateral one and a half toes.
  Muscular: the medial plantar nerve supplies abductor hallucis, flexor hallucis brevis, flexor digitorum brevis and the first lumbrical; the lateral plantar nerve supplies all the other small muscles of the sole.
  For details of nerve branches, see pp. 152 and 153.
- The skin under the heel and on the lateral part of the sole is part of the first sacral dermatome, with the fifth lumbar dermatome including the rest of the sole (**Fig. 9**, p. 153).
- The superficial surface of the plantar aponeurosis is not smooth as in most textbook drawings, but roughened by the attachment of numerous fibrous septa forming loculations that hold the fatty subcutaneous tissues and skin in place when weight-bearing. They are well shown toward the back and sides of the dissection illustrated here.

1 Plantar digital nerve
2 Superficial transverse metatarsal ligament
3 Superficial layer ⎫ of digital band of aponeurosis
4 Deep layer ⎭
5 Transverse fibres of aponeurosis
6 Proper plantar digital nerve of great toe
7 Common plantar digital branch of medial plantar nerve
8 Common plantar digital branch of lateral plantar nerve
9 Central part of aponeurosis overlying flexor digitorum brevis
10 Medial part of aponeurosis overlying abductor hallucis
11 Lateral part of aponeurosis overlying abductor digiti minimi
12 Medial calcanean nerve
13 Medial process of tuberosity of calcaneus
14 Proper plantar digital nerve of fifth toe

Sole of the foot *First layer structures*

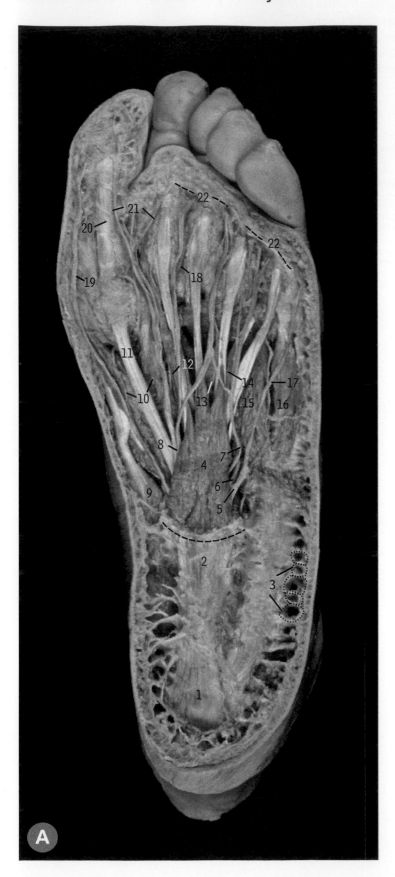

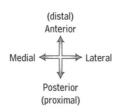

A

The plantar aponeurosis (2):
- Extends from the medial and lateral tubercles of the calcaneus
- Divides at the distal end and forms five slips at the front, one slip for each toe
- Fuses with the fibrous flexor sheaths and metatarsophalangeal joint capsules
- Helps to preserve the longitudinal arches of the foot

The medial plantar nerve (8):
- Supplies the medial part of the side of the foot and the medial three and a half toes

The lateral plantar nerve (5):
- Supplies the lateral part of the sole of foot and lateral one and a half toes

1   Medial process of tuberosity of calcaneus
2   Central part of plantar aponeurosis
3   Fibrous septi forming loculations
4   Flexor digitorum brevis
5   Lateral plantar nerve
6   Lateral plantar artery
7   Fourth common plantar digital nerve
8   Medial plantar nerve
9   Abductor hallucis
10 Flexor hallucis brevis
11 Flexor hallucis longus
12 First ⎫
13 Third ⎬ lumbrical
14 Fourth ⎭
15 Flexor digiti minimi brevis
16 Abductor digiti minimi
17 Proper plantar digital nerve of fifth toe
18 Superficial digital branch of medial plantar artery
19 Proper plantar digital nerve of great toe
20 Fibrous flexor sheath
21 Proper plantar digital nerves of first cleft
22 Superficial transverse metatarsal ligament

(distal)
Anterior

Medial ⟷ Lateral

Posterior
(proximal)

Lower leg and sole of foot

Deep medial structures and second layer from the right and slightly below

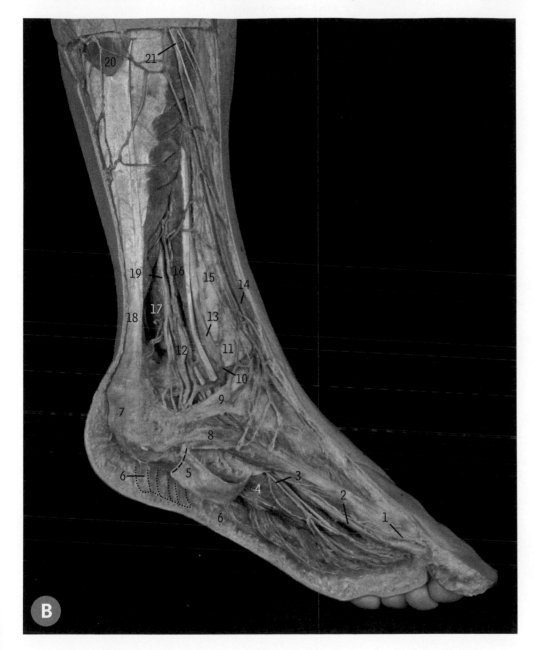

(distal)
Anterior

Med ← → Lat

Posterior
(proximal)

1. Proper plantar digital nerve of great toe
2. Tendon of flexor hallucis longus
3. Medial plantar nerve
4. Flexor digitorum brevis
5. Plantar aponeurosis (reflected superiorly)
6. Dense subcutaneous fatty tissue of sole of foot within fibrous septi (loculations)
7. Posterior surface of calcaneus
8. Abductor hallucis
9. Flexor retinaculum
10. Dorsal venous arch
11. Medial malleolus of tibia
12. Posterior tibial artery and veins
13. Tibialis posterior
14. Great saphenous vein
15. Medial surface of tibia
16. Flexor digitorum longus
17. Flexor hallucis longus
18. Tendo calcaneus (Achilles tendon)
19. Tibial nerve
20. Gastrocnemius
21. Medial branch of superficial fibular (peroneal) nerve

The tendo calcaneus (Achilles tendon) (18):
- Is the thickest tendon in the body and receives muscle fibres from both gastrocnemius and soleus
- Inserts into the middle of the back of the calcaneus
- May be tested for ankle jerk just above its insertion into the calcaneus
- Under excessive exertion is prone to tear (rupture) usually above its insertion into calcaneus, producing a palpable gap as fibres of the tendon 'roll-up' like a window roller blind

The posterior tibial artery (12):
- Can be palpated behind the medial malleolus of the tibia approximately 2.5 cm in front of the medial border of the tendo calcaneus (Achilles tendon) (18)

The great saphenous vein (14):
- Runs in front of the medial malleolus of the tibia

The small saphenous vein:
- Runs behind the lateral malleolus of the fibula

Sole of the foot

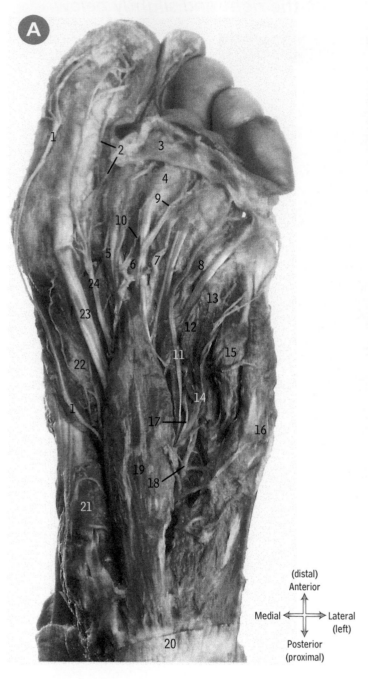

Medial ⟷ Lateral (left)

(distal)
Anterior

Posterior
(proximal)

The plantar aponeurosis has been removed. The central muscle is flexor digitorum brevis (19), with abductor hallucis (21) on the medial side and abductor digiti minimi (16) on the lateral side. The most prominent tendon is that of flexor hallucis longus (23). Digital branches of the medial and lateral plantar nerves (1, 2, 10, 11 and 14) run forward toward the toes, and the deep branch of the lateral plantar nerve (17), which supplies many of the deeper muscles, curves deeply into the sole. See also Fig. 4, p. 150.

- The muscles of the sole are usually classified in **four layers**, as seen in progressively deep dissection:
  First layer: abductor hallucis (**A21**), flexor digitorum brevis (**A19**) and abductor digiti minimi (**A16**).
  Second layer: Quadratus plantae (**B19**) and the four lumbrical muscles (**B7–10**), with the tendons of flexor digitorum longus (**B4**) and flexor hallucis longus (**B1**).
  Third layer: flexor hallucis brevis (p. 94, **A8**), adductor hallucis (p. 94, **A6** and **7**) and flexor digiti minimi brevis (p. 94, **A14**).
  Fourth layer: three plantar and four dorsal interosseus muscles (p. 95, **B5–11**), with the tendons of tibialis posterior (p. 95, **B27**) and fibularis (*peroneus*) longus (p. 95, **B24**).
  The successive layers do not completely obscure one another; for example, the third plantar and fourth dorsal interossei (**A13** and **12**) are seen as soon as the plantar aponeurosis has been removed. (The layers refer to layers of *muscles*; the plantar aponeurosis is not itself the first layer but overlies it.)
- It may be functionally more useful to classify the muscles into **medial**, **lateral** and **intermediate** groups:
  Medial group, for the great toe: abductor hallucis, flexor hallucis brevis, adductor hallucis and the tendon of flexor hallucis longus
  Lateral group, for the fifth toe: abductor digiti minimi and flexor digiti minimi brevis
  Intermediate group, for the second to fifth toes: flexor digitorum brevis, quadratus plantae, the tendons of flexor digitorum longus and the lumbricals, and the interossei

1 Proper plantar digital nerve of great toe	**13** Third plantar interosseus
2 Proper plantar digital nerves of first cleft	**14** Proper plantar digital nerve of fifth toe
3 Superficial transverse metatarsal ligament	**15** Flexor digiti minimi brevis
4 Fibrous flexor sheath	**16** Abductor digiti minimi
5 First lumbrical	**17** Deep branch of lateral plantar nerve
6 Second lumbrical	**18** Lateral plantar artery
7 Third lumbrical	**19** Flexor digitorum brevis
8 Fourth lumbrical	**20** Plantar aponeurosis
9 Third plantar metatarsal artery	**21** Abductor hallucis
10 A superficial digital branch of medial plantar artery	**22** Flexor hallucis brevis
11 Fourth common plantar digital nerve	**23** Flexor hallucis longus
12 Fourth dorsal interosseus	**24** First common plantar digital nerve

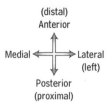

B Second layer of muscles of the left sole

Flexor digitorum brevis has been removed (but the abductors of the great and little toes, 27 and 16, remain) to display quadratus plantae (19) joining flexor digitorum longus (4) as it divides into its four tendons, from which the lumbrical muscles arise (7–10). The deep branch of the lateral plantar nerve (18) curls round the lateral side of quadratus plantae (19) to reach the deeper part of the sole, and numerous other muscular and digital (cutaneous) branches of the medial and lateral plantar nerves (26 and 22) are visible. Synovial sheaths of flexor tendons have been emphasized by blue tissue. See also Fig. 5, p. 150.

- Although flexor hallucis longus (**B1**) passes to the great toe on the *medial* side of the foot, it arises from the *fibula* on the lateral side of the leg. The tendon crosses over in the sole, deep to flexor digitorum longus (**B4**, toward the back of the sole).
- The lateral and medial plantar nerves and vessels (**B20, 22** and **26**) pass between the first and second layers of muscles. The deep branch of the lateral plantar nerve (**A17, B18**) and the deep branch of the artery, which becomes the lateral plantar arch (**B17**), curl deeply round the lateral border of quadratus plantae (**B19**).

1 Flexor hallucis longus
2 Fibrous flexor sheath
3 Flexor digitorum brevis
4 Flexor digitorum longus
5 Proper plantar digital nerve of great toe
6 Flexor hallucis brevis
7 First lumbrical
8 Second lumbrical
9 Third lumbrical
10 Fourth lumbrical
11 Fourth plantar metatarsal artery
12 Fourth dorsal interosseus
13 Third plantar interosseus
14 Proper plantar digital nerve of fifth toe
15 Flexor digiti minimi brevis
16 Abductor digiti minimi
17 Plantar arch
18 Deep branch of lateral plantar nerve
19 Quadratus plantae
20 Lateral plantar artery
21 Nerve to abductor digiti minimi
22 Lateral plantar nerve
23 Fourth common plantar digital nerve
24 Nerve to quadratus plantae
25 Nerve to flexor digitorum brevis
26 Medial plantar artery overlying nerve
27 Abductor hallucis
28 Nerve to flexor hallucis brevis
29 First common plantar digital nerve
30 Nerve to first lumbrical

(distal)
Anterior

Medial ←→ Lateral
(left)

Posterior
(proximal)

Sole of the foot

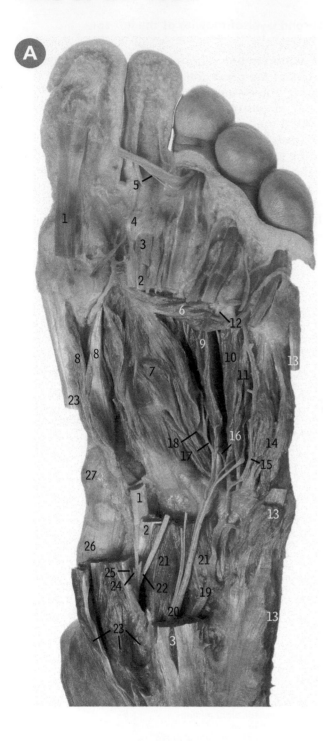

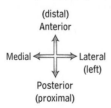

(distal)
Anterior

Medial ⟷ Lateral
(left)

Posterior
(proximal)

A Third layer of muscles of the left sole

Most of the flexors and abductors have been removed, displaying the two heads of adductor hallucis (6 and 7), flexor hallucis brevis (8, which divides to pass to either side of the great toe), flexor digiti minimi brevis (14) and interossei (9–11). The deep branch of the lateral plantar nerve (17) is accompanied by the plantar arch (16) (from the lateral plantar artery, 19). See also Fig. 6, p. 151.

- For a summary of the medial and lateral plantar nerves, see p. 153.
- The third common plantar digital nerve (from the medial plantar nerve) frequently has a communicating branch with the (fourth) common plantar digital branch of the lateral plantar nerve, but it was not present in the specimens dissected here.
- Branches of the lateral plantar nerve (**A20, B21**) to various interosseus muscles (**A9–11, B5–11**) can be seen but have been left unlabeled.
- The plantar arch (**B18**) is the deep continuation of the lateral plantar artery (**B20**), which is the larger terminal branch of the posterior tibial artery. The arch is completed by anastomosis with the deep plantar (perforating) branch of the first dorsal metatarsal artery (see p. 84, **15**).
  The arch gives off four plantar metatarsal arteries (as in **B15** and **16**), which divide to give plantar digital branches to the sides of adjacent toes. There are separate branches for the medial side of the great toe and lateral side of the fifth toe.
- The medial plantar artery (**A24, B23**), smaller than the lateral and subject to considerable variation, does not take part directly in the formation of the arch. It usually anastomoses with the plantar digital branch to the medial side of the great toe, and gives off superficial digital branches that anastomose with the first three plantar metatarsal arteries.

1 Flexor hallucis longus
2 Flexor digitorum longus
3 Flexor digitorum brevis
4 Fibrous flexor sheath
5 Long vinculum
6 Transverse head ⎫ of adductor hallucis
7 Oblique head ⎭
8 Flexor hallucis brevis
9 Second plantar interosseus
10 Fourth dorsal interosseus
11 Third plantar interosseus
12 Fourth plantar metatarsal artery
13 Abductor digiti minimi
14 Flexor digiti minimi brevis
15 Nerve to flexor digiti minimi brevis
16 Plantar arch
17 Deep branch of lateral plantar nerve
18 Nerve to adductor hallucis
19 Lateral plantar artery
20 Lateral plantar nerve
21 Quadratus plantae
22 Medial plantar nerve
23 Abductor hallucis
24 Medial plantar artery
25 Nerve to abductor hallucis
26 Tuberosity of navicular
27 Tibialis anterior

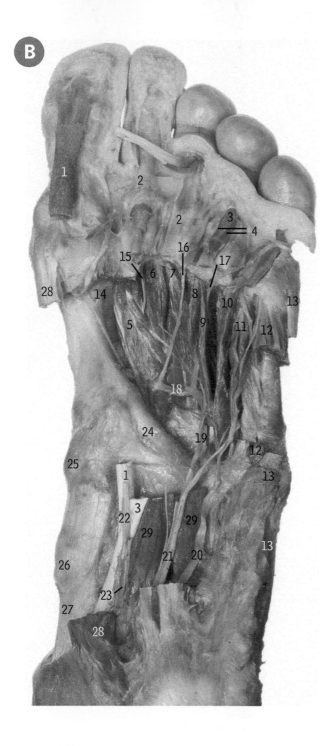

B

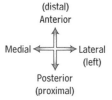

(distal)
Anterior

Medial ← → Lateral
(left)

Posterior
(proximal)

B Fourth layer of muscles of the left sole

Most of the smaller muscles have been removed, leaving only the three plantar interossei (7, 9 and 11) and the four dorsal interossei (5, 6, 8 and 10). The tendon of tibialis posterior (27) passes mainly to the tuberosity of the navicular (26), and the tendon of fibularis (peroneus) longus (24) crosses the sole obliquely from the lateral to the medial side. The end of the synovial sheath of flexor hallucis longus (1) has been emphasized by blue tissue. See also Fig. 7, p. 151.

- Viewed from the sole, both plantar *and* dorsal interossei (**B5–11**) are visible; they lie side by side, not (as might be expected from their names) with the plantar group completely overlying and obscuring the dorsal. (But, on the dorsum only dorsal interossei are seen between the metatarsals—as on p. 80, **A15–18**.)
  The *plantar* interossei *ad*duct toes and the *dorsal* interossei *ab*duct them at the metatarsophalangeal joints, the reference line or axis for these movements being the line of the second toe. The mnemonics PAD and DAB are the usual aids to recalling which group does what.
  The great toe and the fifth toe each have their own abductor muscle; the great toe also has its own adductor to draw it nearer the second toe. It follows that there must be a plantar interosseus for each of the third, fourth and fifth toes so that they can be adducted toward the axial line. The second toe has no plantar interosseus, but it has two dorsal interossei, one on each side so that it can be abducted to either side of its own neutral position. The third and fourth toes both have one of each interosseus.
- For other and probably more important actions of the interossei, see p. 107.
- For a summary of the medial and lateral plantar arteries, see p. 169.

1 Flexor hallucis longus
2 Fibrous flexor sheath
3 Flexor digitorum longus
4 Flexor digitorum brevis
5 First dorsal ⎫
6 Second dorsal ⎪
7 First plantar ⎪
8 Third dorsal ⎬ interosseus
9 Second plantar ⎪
10 Fourth dorsal ⎪
11 Third plantar ⎭
12 Flexor digiti minimi brevis
13 Abductor digiti minimi
14 First plantar metatarsal artery
15 Second plantar metatarsal artery
16 Third plantar metatarsal artery
17 Fourth plantar metatarsal artery
18 Plantar arch
19 Deep branch of lateral plantar nerve
20 Lateral plantar artery
21 Lateral ⎫ plantar nerve
22 Medial ⎭
23 Medial plantar artery
24 Fibularis (peroneus) longus
25 Tibialis anterior
26 Tuberosity of navicular
27 Tibialis posterior
28 Abductor hallucis
29 Quadratus plantae

Ligaments of the foot *Ligaments of the right foot*

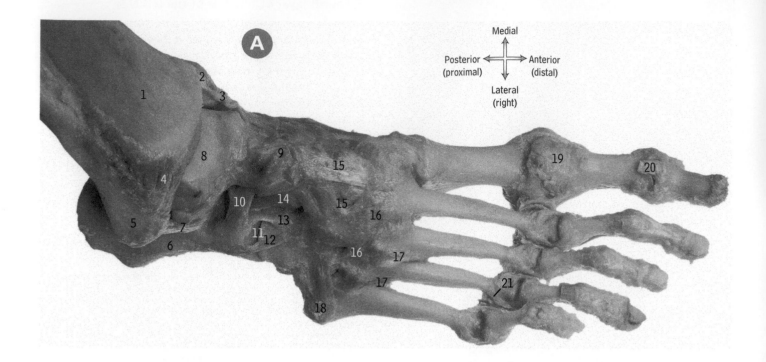

Medial
Posterior ← → Anterior
(proximal)　(distal)
Lateral
(right)

A

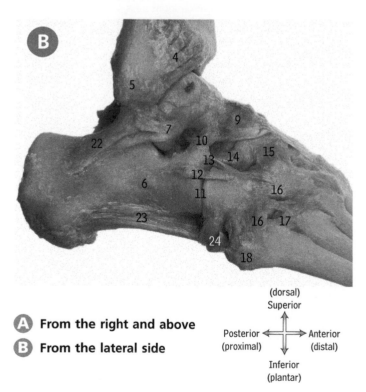

B

(dorsal)
Superior
Posterior ← → Anterior
(proximal)　(distal)
Inferior
(plantar)

A From the right and above
B From the lateral side

 1　Tibia
 2　Medial malleolus
 3　Medial (deltoid) ligament of ankle joint
 4　Anterior tibiofibular ligament
 5　Lateral malleolus
 6　Calcaneus
 7　Anterior talofibular ligament
 8　Trochlear surface of talus (ankle joint capsule removed)
 9　Head of talus (under capsule of talonavicular part of talocalcaneonavicular joint)
10　Cervical ligament
11　Calcaneocuboid joint
12　Dorsal calcaneocuboid ligament
13　Calcaneocuboid part
14　Calcaneonavicular part　} of bifurcate ligament
15　Dorsal cuneonavicular ligaments
16　Dorsal tarsometatarsal ligaments
17　Dorsal metatarsal ligaments
18　Tuberosity of base of fifth metatarsal
19　Capsule of first metatarsophalangeal joint
20　Tendon of extensor hallucis longus
21　Collateral ligament
22　Calcaneofibular ligament
23　Long plantar ligament
24　Tendon of fibularis (*peroneus*) longus
25　Interosseous membrane
26　Posterior tibiofibular ligament
27　Tibial slip of 28
28　Posterior talofibular ligament
29　Groove for flexor hallucis longus tendon on talus and sustentaculum tali
30　Posterior tibiotalar part
31　Tibiocalcanean part (deltoid)　} of medial deltoid ligament
32　Groove for tibialis posterior tendon
33　Groove for fibularis (*peroneus*) brevis tendon

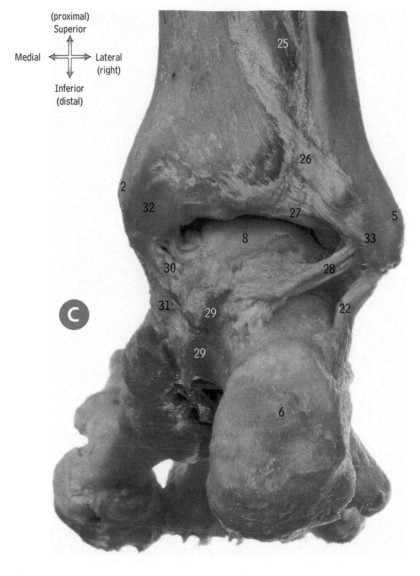

(proximal)
Superior

Medial ←→ Lateral
(right)

Inferior
(distal)

25

26

2

32

27

5

8

33

30

28

31

29

22

29

6

C From behind

In A the foot is plantarflexed, showing part of the trochlear (superior articular) surface of the talus (8), with the front of the deltoid ligament (3) on the medial side and the anterior tibiofibular ligament (4) on the lateral side. The cervical ligament (10) passes upward and medially from the upper surface of the calcaneus to the undersurface of the talus, and in front of it are the two parts of the bifurcate ligament (13 and 14) with a small dorsal calcaneocuboid ligament (12) more laterally. Other dorsal ligaments (15, 16 and 17) connect adjacent bones.

In B the anterior talofibular ligament (7) and calcaneofibular ligament (22) are seen, with some of the smaller dorsal ligaments (12–17), and so is the posterior part of the long plantar ligament (23) in the sole.

In C the posterior talofibular ligament (28) runs transversely (so it is not seen in the lateral view in B); it has a tibial slip (27), which merges with the inferior transverse ligament, the name given to the lower part of the posterior tibiofibular ligament (26).

- On the medial side of the ankle joint there is a single medial (deltoid) ligament (**A3**) (although it has several parts, as on p. 98, **A2–5**), but on the lateral side there is no single lateral ligament but three separate ligaments: the anterior and posterior talofibular ligaments (**A7** and **B7**, **C28**) and the calcaneofibular ligament (**B22** and **C22**).

Ligaments of the foot

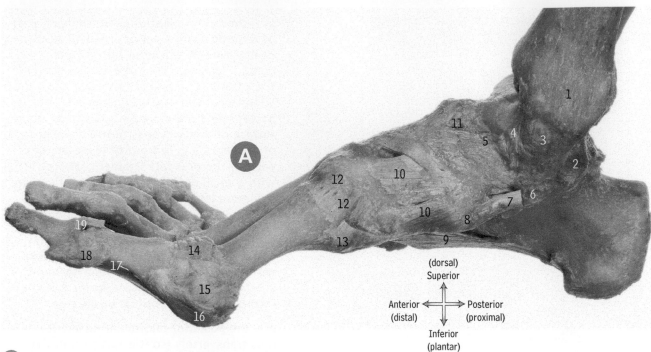

On the medial side of the ankle the various parts of the medial (deltoid) ligament (2–5) merge with one another. The tendon of tibialis posterior (7) is mainly attached to the tuberosity of the navicular (8), while that of tibialis anterior (13) runs to the medial cuneiform and the base of the first metatarsal.

1 Medial malleolus
2 Posterior tibiotalar part ⎫
3 Tibiocalcanean part   ⎬ of medial (deltoid) ligament
4 Anterior tibiotalar part ⎪
5 Tibionavicular part   ⎭
6 Sustentaculum tali
7 Tibialis posterior
8 Tuberosity of navicular
9 Long plantar ligament
10 Dorsal cuneonavicular ligament
11 Talonavicular ligament
12 Dorsal ligaments of first tarsometatarsal joint
13 Tibialis anterior
14 Capsule   ⎫ of first metatarsophalangeal joint
15 Collateral ligament ⎭
16 Sesamoid bone
17 Flexor hallucis longus
18 Collateral ligament of interphalangeal joint
19 Extensor hallucis longus

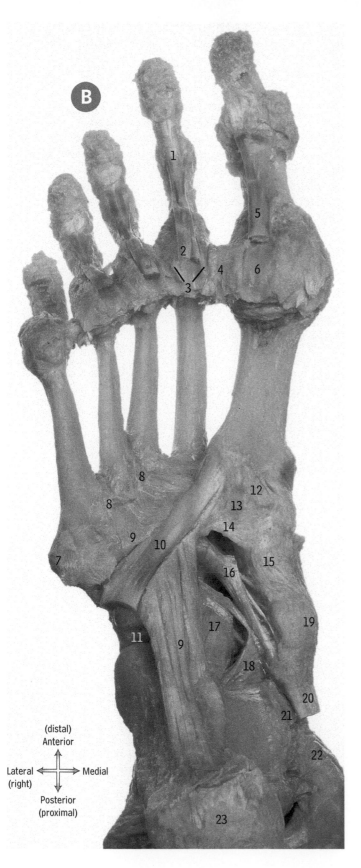

(distal)
Anterior

Lateral ←→ Medial
(right)

Posterior
(proximal)

B Ligaments of the sole of the right foot

Part of the long plantar ligament (9) has been cut away to show the tendon of fibularis (*peroneus*) longus (10) lying in the groove on the cuboid. Medial to the posterior part of the long plantar ligament is the short plantar (plantar calcaneocuboid) ligament (17), and medial to that is the spring (plantar calcaneonavicular) ligament (18). At the anterior part of the foot the deep transverse metatarsal ligaments (4) keep the heads of the metatarsals and the bases of the toes from spreading apart.

 1 Flexor digitorum longus
 2 Flexor digitorum brevis
 3 Fibrous flexor sheath
 4 Deep transverse metatarsal ligament
 5 Flexor hallucis longus
 6 Plantar ligament of first tarsometatarsal joint
 7 Tuberosity of base of fifth metatarsal
 8 Plantar metatarsal ligaments
 9 Long plantar ligament
10 Tendon of fibularis *(peroneus)* longus in groove on cuboid
11 Calcaneocuboid joint
12 Plantar tarsometatarsal ligament
13 Medial cuneiform
14 Cuneometatarsal ligament
15 Plantar cuneonavicular ligament
16 Fibrous slip from tibialis posterior overlying a cuneometatarsal ligament
17 Plantar calcaneocuboid (short plantar) ligament
18 Plantar calcaneonavicular (spring) ligament
19 Tuberosity of navicular
20 Tendon of tibialis posterior
21 Sustentaculum tali and groove for flexor hallucis longus
22 Medial (deltoid) ligament of ankle joint
23 Tuberosity of calcaneus

- The *medial* sides of the medial cuneiform and the base of the first metatarsal receive the attachment of the tibialis anterior tendon (**A13**); the *lateral* sides of the same two bones receive the attachment of the fibularis *(peroneus)* longus tendon (**B10**).
- The plantar calcaneocuboid ligament (**B17**), commonly called the short plantar ligament, is largely under cover of the long plantar ligament (**B9**), which with the groove on the cuboid bone forms an osseofibrous tunnel for the fibularis *(peroneus)* longus tendon (**B10**).
- The plantar calcaneonavicular ligament (**B18**), passing from the sustentaculum tali of the calcaneus to the navicular and commonly called the spring ligament although it is not elastic, is an important support for the head of the talus in the talocalcaneonavicular joint (p. 87, **15**).

Sections of the foot *Sagittal sections of the right foot*

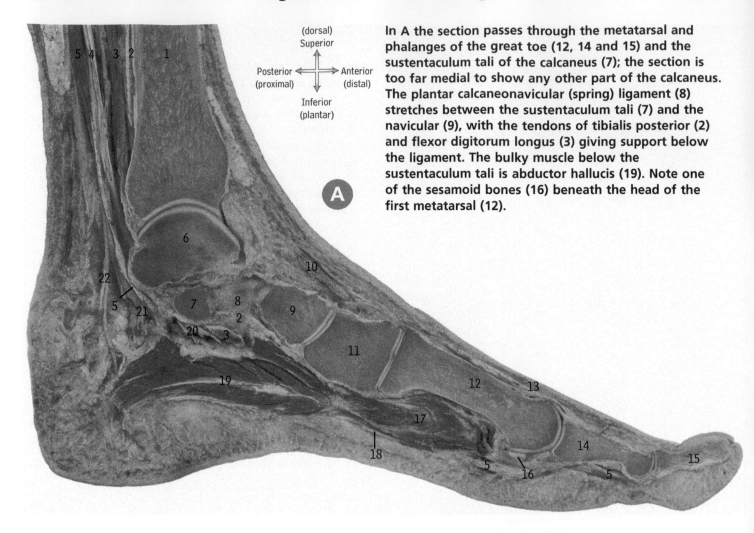

(dorsal)
Superior

Posterior ⟵ ⟶ Anterior
(proximal)   (distal)

Inferior
(plantar)

In A the section passes through the metatarsal and phalanges of the great toe (12, 14 and 15) and the sustentaculum tali of the calcaneus (7); the section is too far medial to show any other part of the calcaneus. The plantar calcaneonavicular (spring) ligament (8) stretches between the sustentaculum tali (7) and the navicular (9), with the tendons of tibialis posterior (2) and flexor digitorum longus (3) giving support below the ligament. The bulky muscle below the sustentaculum tali is abductor hallucis (19). Note one of the sesamoid bones (16) beneath the head of the first metatarsal (12).

A   Through the medial part of the talus, sustentaculum tali of the calcaneus and the great toe, from the lateral side

1 Tibia	**11** Medial cuneiform
2 Tibialis posterior	**12** First metatarsal
3 Flexor digitorum longus	**13** Extensor hallucis longus
4 Tibial nerve	**14** Proximal phalanx
5 Flexor hallucis longus	**15** Distal phalanx
6 Talus	**16** Sesamoid bone
7 Sustentaculum tali	**17** Flexor hallucis brevis
8 Plantar calcaneonavicular (spring) ligament	**18** Proper plantar digital nerve of great toe
9 Navicular	**19** Abductor hallucis
10 Tibialis anterior	**20** Medial plantar nerve and vessels

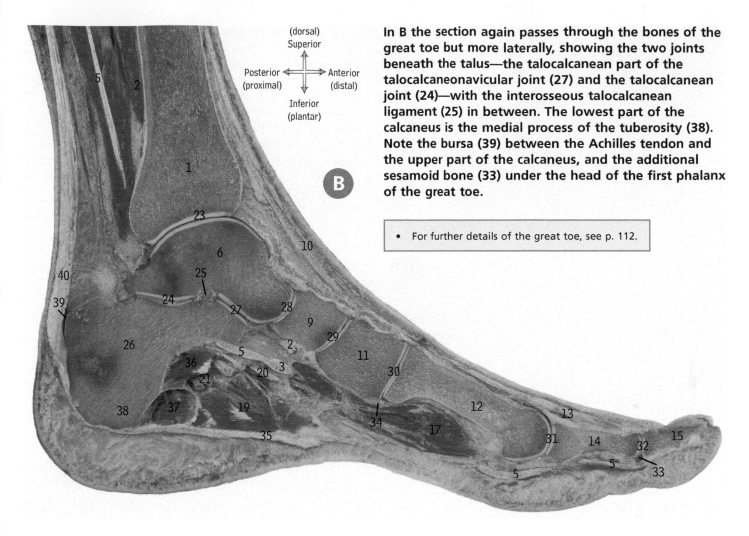

In B the section again passes through the bones of the great toe but more laterally, showing the two joints beneath the talus—the talocalcanean part of the talocalcaneonavicular joint (27) and the talocalcanean joint (24)—with the interosseous talocalcanean ligament (25) in between. The lowest part of the calcaneus is the medial process of the tuberosity (38). Note the bursa (39) between the Achilles tendon and the upper part of the calcaneus, and the additional sesamoid bone (33) under the head of the first phalanx of the great toe.

• For further details of the great toe, see p. 112.

B **Through the center of the talus, medial part of the calcaneus and the great toe, from the lateral side (in a different foot from that in A)**

21 Lateral plantar nerve and vessels
22 Medial calcanean nerve
23 Ankle joint
24 Talocalcanean joint
25 Interosseous talocalcanean ligament
26 Calcaneus
27 Talocalcanean part } of talocalcaneonavicular joint
28 Talonavicular part
29 Cuneonavicular joint
30 Cuneometatarsal joint

31 Metatarsophalangeal joint
32 Interphalangeal joint
33 Additional sesamoid bone
34 Fibularis (peroneus) longus
35 Plantar aponeurosis
36 Quadratus plantae
37 Abductor digiti minimi
38 Medial process of tuberosity of calcaneus
39 Bursa
40 Tendo calcaneus

Sections of the foot *Sagittal sections of the right foot*

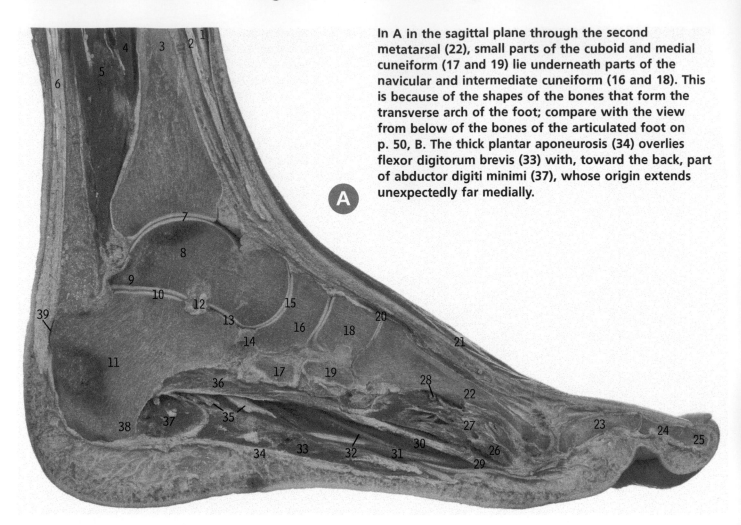

In A in the sagittal plane through the second metatarsal (22), small parts of the cuboid and medial cuneiform (17 and 19) lie underneath parts of the navicular and intermediate cuneiform (16 and 18). This is because of the shapes of the bones that form the transverse arch of the foot; compare with the view from below of the bones of the articulated foot on p. 50, B. The thick plantar aponeurosis (34) overlies flexor digitorum brevis (33) with, toward the back, part of abductor digiti minimi (37), whose origin extends unexpectedly far medially.

A Through the second toe, from the lateral side

1 Tibialis anterior	**11** Calcaneus
2 Extensor hallucis longus	**12** Interosseous talocalcanean ligament
3 Tibia	**13** Talocalcanean part of talocalcaneonavicular joint
4 Tibialis posterior	**14** Plantar calcaneonavicular (spring) ligament
5 Flexor hallucis longus	**15** Talonavicular part of talocalcaneonavicular joint
6 Tendo calcaneus	**16** Navicular
7 Ankle joint	**17** Cuboid
8 Talus	**18** Intermediate cuneiform
9 Lateral tubercle of talus	**19** Medial cuneiform
10 Talocalcanean joint	**20** Extensor digitorum brevis

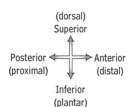

(dorsal) Superior — Posterior (proximal) / Anterior (distal) — Inferior (plantar)

In B through the sagittal plane of the fifth metatarsal (47), the tendon of fibularis (*peroneus*) longus (42) is seen coursing obliquely under the cuboid (17); compare with 10 on p. 98.

21 Extensor digitorum longus tendon to second toe
22 Second metatarsal
23 Proximal
24 Middle } phalanx of second toe
25 Distal
26 Transverse head } of adductor hallucis
27 Oblique head
28 Plantar arch
29 Second lumbrical overlying flexor digitorum longus
   tendon to second toe
30 Flexor digitorum longus tendon to third toe
31 Flexor digitorum brevis tendon to second toe
32 Second common plantar digital nerve
33 Flexor digitorum brevis
34 Plantar aponeurosis
35 Lateral plantar nerve and vessels
36 Quadratus plantae
37 Abductor digiti minimi
38 Medial process of tuberosity of calcaneus
39 Bursa
40 Lateral branch of superficial fibular (*peroneal*)
   nerve
41 Fibula
42 Fibularis (*peroneus*) longus
43 Fibularis (*peroneus*) brevis
44 Lateral process of tuberosity of calcaneus
45 Calcaneocuboid joint
46 Cuboideometatarsal joint
47 Fifth metatarsal
48 Flexor digiti minimi brevis
49 Metatarsophalangeal joint of fifth toe

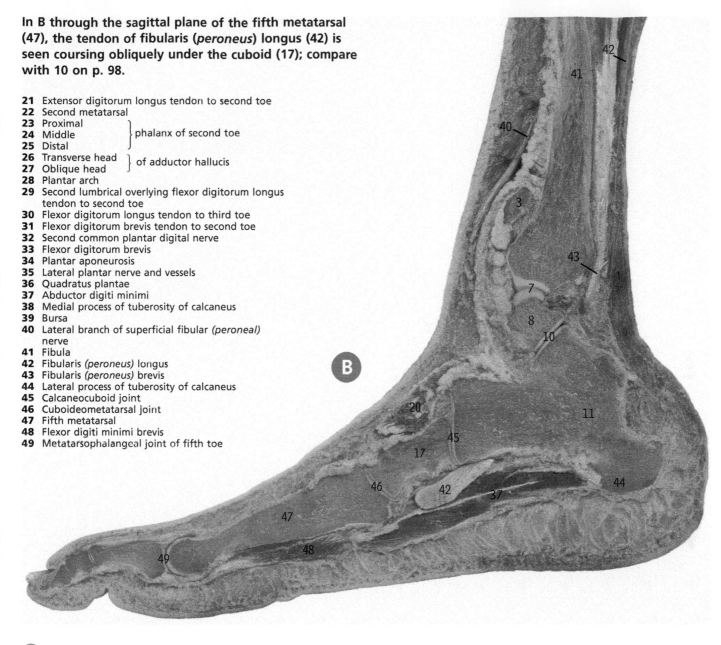

B Through the fifth toe, from the medial side

(dorsal)
Superior

Anterior ←→ Posterior
(distal)   (proximal)

Inferior
(plantar)

Sections of the foot

Axial sections and images of the right lower leg and foot

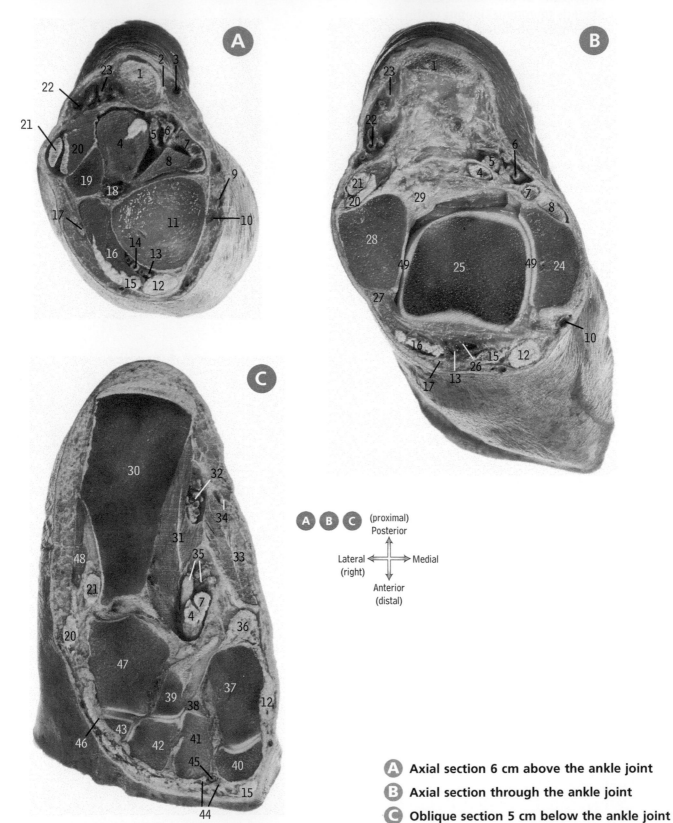

A Axial section 6 cm above the ankle joint

B Axial section through the ankle joint

C Oblique section 5 cm below the ankle joint

Above the ankle in A, fibularis (*peroneus*) brevis (20) is behind the fibula (19) with the tendon of fibularis (*peroneus*) longus (21) lying laterally, but at the lower levels in B and C the tendon of fibularis (*peroneus*) longus (21) is behind that of fibularis (*peroneus*) brevis (20). The lowest part of flexor hallucis longus (4) is seen arising from the fibula (19).

At the level of the medial malleolus (24) in B, the tendon of tibialis posterior (8) lies adjacent to the bone, with the tendon of flexor digitorum longus (7) immediately behind it. The posterior tibial vessels (6) and the tibial nerve (5) intervene between the flexor digitorum tendon (7) and the tendon of flexor hallucis longus (4). At the front of the medial malleolus (24) in B, note the great saphenous vein (10), and in front of

the talus (25) the dorsalis pedis artery (26) and deep fibular (*peroneal*) nerve (13) lie between the tendons of extensor hallucis longus (15) and extensor digitorum longus (16).

In the oblique section in C, the cuboid (47) lies in front of the calcaneus (30), and at a lower level the tendon of fibularis (*peroneus*) longus (21) will pass underneath the cuboid. On the medial side behind the medial cuneiform (37), the very tip of the tuberosity of the navicular (36) receives the main attachment of tibialis posterior. The tendons of flexor hallucis longus (4) and flexor digitorum longus (7) are more laterally placed.

The sections A, B and C are viewed from above, looking from the knee toward the ankle.

1 Tendo calcaneus
2 Plantaris
3 A tributary of great saphenous vein
4 Flexor hallucis longus
5 Tibial nerve
6 Posterior tibial vessels
7 Flexor digitorum longus
8 Tibialis posterior
9 Saphenous nerve
10 Great saphenous vein
11 Tibia
12 Tibialis anterior
13 Deep fibular (*peroneal*) nerve
14 Anterior tibial vessels
15 Extensor hallucis longus
16 Extensor digitorum longus
17 Superficial fibular (*peroneal*) nerve
18 Fibular (*peroneal*) vessels
19 Fibula
20 Fibularis (*peroneus*) brevis
21 Fibularis (*peroneus*) longus
22 Small saphenous vein
23 Sural nerve
24 Medial malleolus
25 Talus

26 Dorsalis pedis artery
27 Anterior talofibular ligament
28 Lateral malleolus
29 Posterior talofibular ligament
30 Calcaneus
31 Quadratus plantae
32 Lateral plantar nerve and vessels
33 Abductor hallucis
34 Medial calcanean nerve
35 Medial plantar nerve and vessels
36 Tip of tuberosity of navicular and tibialis posterior
37 Medial ⎫
38 Intermediate ⎬ cuneiform
39 Lateral ⎭
40 First ⎫
41 Second ⎬ metatarsal base
42 Third
43 Fourth ⎭
44 First dorsal interosseus
45 Deep plantar artery
46 Extensor digitorum brevis
47 Cuboid
48 Abductor digiti minimi
49 Ankle joint

Sections of the foot

Coronal sections of the left ankle joint and foot (in plantarflexion)

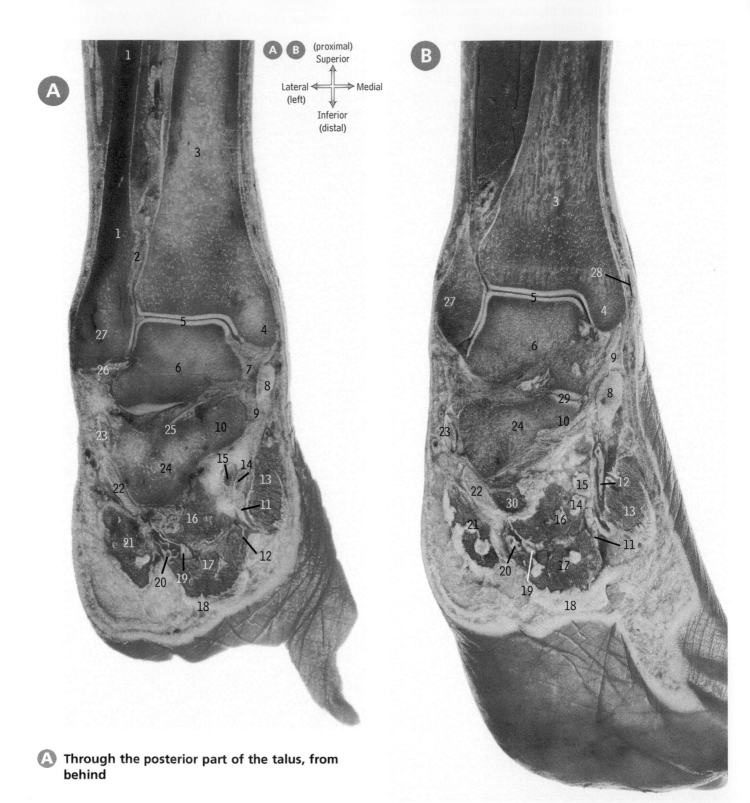

A Through the posterior part of the talus, from behind

B About 1 cm in front of A, through the talocalcanean part of the talocalcaneonavicular joint, from behind

These coronal sections through the ankle joint (5) emphasize how the talus (6) is gripped between the two malleoli (27 and 4). In A the interosseous talocalcanean ligament (25) lies between the talus (6) and calcaneus (24), while in B the section has passed through the part of the sustentaculum tali (10), which forms the talocalcanean part of the talocalcaneonavicular joint (29). In the center of the sole in both sections, flexor digitorum brevis (17) overlies quadratus plantae (16); the fusion of plantae with the tendon of flexor digitorum longus (14) is shown in B, where the tendon of flexor hallucis longus (15) has come to lie deep to the digitorum tendon (compare with the dissection B on p. 93 and the section B on p. 110).

- Joints, muscles and movements:
  At the ankle joint
  Dorsiflexion: tibialis anterior, extensor hallucis longus, extensor digitorum longus and fibularis (*peroneus*) tertius
  Plantarflexion: gastrocnemius, soleus, plantaris, tibialis posterior, flexor hallucis longus and flexor digitorum longus
  At the talocalcanean and talocalcaneonavicular joints
  Inversion: tibialis anterior and tibialis posterior
  Eversion: fibularis (*peroneus*) longus, fibularis (*peroneus*) brevis and fibularis (*peroneus*) tertius
- At the other small joints of the foot there are minor degrees of gliding or rotatory movements. At the transverse tarsal joint (p. 57) a small amount of inversion and eversion occurs, but by far the greater part of these important movements takes place at the two joints beneath the talus. To visualize inversion and eversion, imagine the talus held firmly between the tibia and fibula, and the whole of the rest of the foot swivelling inwards or outwards underneath the talus. These movements do not take place at the ankle joint, which essentially only allows dorsiflexion and plantarflexion.
- The actions of muscles on the toes are indicated by their names, but the part played by the interossei and lumbricals requires some explanation (apart from the abduction and adduction produced by the interossei and referred to on p. 95). Briefly the interossei and lumbricals work together to flex the metatarsophalangeal joints and extend the interphalangeal joints; these apparently contradictory actions on different joints by the same muscles can be explained as follows.
- The interossei (both plantar and dorsal) are attached mainly to the sides of the proximal phalanges but also into the dorsal digital expansions; the lumbricals are usually attached entirely to the expansions. Because of the position of these attachments in relation to the axis of movement of the metatarsophalangeal joints, the interossei and lumbricals plantarflex these joints.
- Because the lumbrical attachments and parts of the interosseus attachments are to the basal angles of the expansions, the line of pull is transmitted to the dorsal surfaces of the toes distal to the metatarsophalangeal joints, and so the interphalangeal joints are extended.
- In most feet the interosseus attachment to the expansion is minimal, and it is the lumbricals that are mainly responsible for assisting the long and short extensor tendons in extending the toes, keeping them straight and stabilized against the pull of the flexors, which tend to make them buckle, especially during the push-off phase of walking when flexor hallucis longus and flexor digitorum longus are contracting strongly.

1 Fibula
2 Interosseous tibiofibular ligament
3 Tibia
4 Medial malleolus
5 Ankle joint
6 Talus
7 Deep part of medial (deltoid) ligament
8 Tibialis posterior
9 Medial ligament
10 Sustentaculum tali
11 Medial plantar nerve
12 Medial plantar artery
13 Abductor hallucis
14 Flexor digitorum longus
15 Flexor hallucis longus
16 Quadratus plantae
17 Flexor digitorum brevis
18 Plantar aponeurosis
19 Lateral plantar nerve
20 Lateral plantar vessels
21 Abductor digiti minimi
22 Fibularis (*peroneus*) longus
23 Fibularis (*peroneus*) brevis
24 Calcaneus
25 Interosseous talocalcanean ligament
26 Posterior talofibular ligament
27 Lateral malleolus
28 Great saphenous vein
29 Talocalcanean part of talocalcaneonavicular joint
30 Cuboid

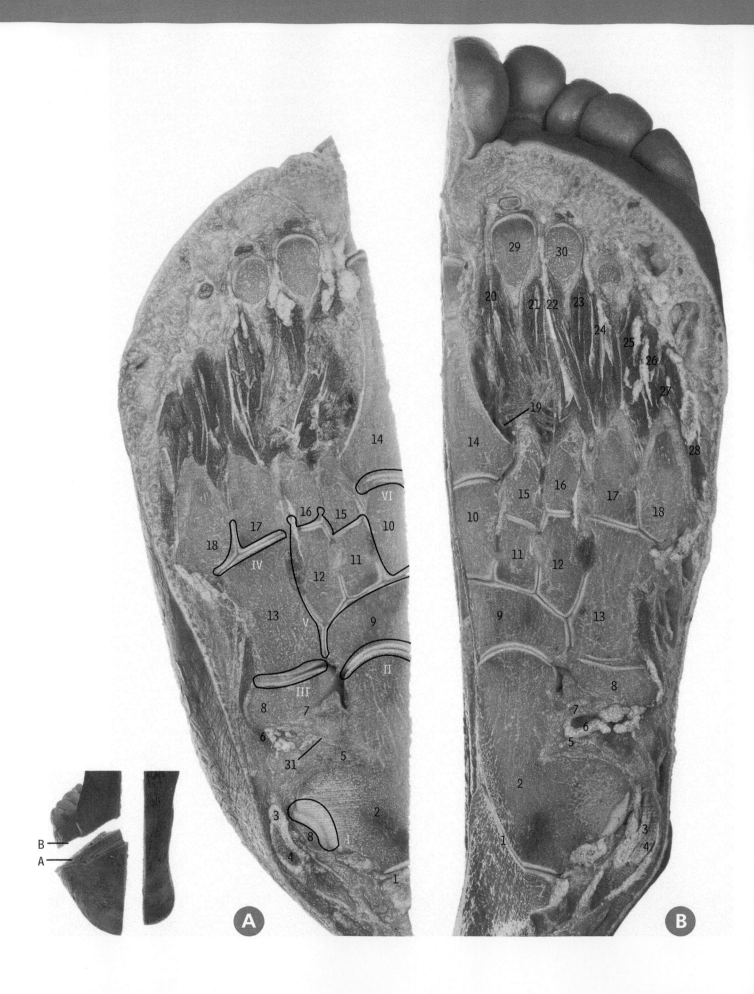

Sections of the foot *Oblique axial sections of the left foot*

The plane of section is shown in the small illustration. The surfaces A and B have been separated and are viewed like two pages in an open book.

Between the tarsal bones in A, the various joint cavities, outlined in black and numbered with Roman figures, are explained in the notes below.

In B the navicular (9) is seen between the talus (2) and the three cuneiforms (10–12). Note how the base of the second metatarsal (15) projects more proximally than the bases of the first and third metatarsals (14 and 16). On the lateral side the cuboid (13) articulates at the back with the very small part of the calcaneus (8) seen in this section, and at the front with the bases of the fourth and fifth metatarsals (17 and 18). Parts of all the interosseus muscles (four dorsal and three plantar, 20–26) are identified in the forefoot.

1 Ankle joint
2 Talus
3 Fibularis (*peroneus*) brevis
4 Fibularis (*peroneus*) longus
5 Interosseous talocalcanean ligament
6 Extensor digitorum brevis
7 Cervical ligament
8 Calcaneus
9 Navicular
10 Medial ⎫
11 Intermediate ⎬ cuneiform
12 Lateral ⎭
13 Cuboid
14 First ⎫
15 Second ⎪
16 Third ⎬ metatarsal base
17 Fourth ⎪
18 Fifth ⎭
19 Deep plantar branch of first dorsal metatarsal artery
20 First dorsal ⎫
21 Second dorsal ⎪
22 First plantar ⎪
23 Third dorsal ⎬ interosseus
24 Second plantar ⎪
25 Fourth dorsal ⎪
26 Third plantar ⎭
27 Flexor digiti minimi brevis
28 Abductor digiti minimi
29 Head of second metatarsal
30 Head of third metatarsal
31 Inferior extensor retinaculum

- The cavities of a number of synovial joints in the foot are continuous with one another to the extent that there are normally six synovial cavities associated with the tarsal bones:
  I The talocalcanean joint cavity
  II The talocalcaneonavicular joint cavity
  III The calcaneocuboid joint cavity
  IV The cuboideometatarsal joint cavity (between the cuboid and the bases of the fourth and fifth metatarsals)
  V The cuneonavicular and cuneometatarsal joint cavity (between the navicular, the three cuneiforms and the bases of the second, third and fourth metatarsals)
  VI The medial cuneometatarsal joint cavity (between the medial cuneiform and the base of the first metatarsal)
- Parts of all the above cavities can be seen in the foot sectioned here; they are indicated by the black lines in **A** and numbered as above. (The cuboideonavicular joint is usually a fibrous union, but in this specimen it is synovial and continuous with the cuneonavicular joint cavity.)

Sections of the foot *Coronal sections of the tarsus of the right foot*

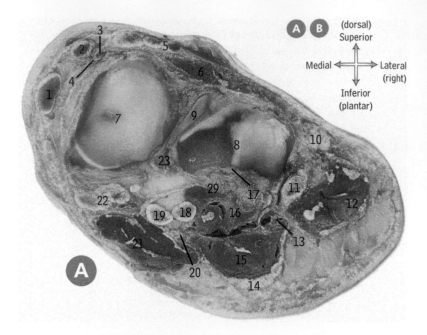

(dorsal) Superior

Medial ◄────► Lateral (right)

Inferior (plantar)

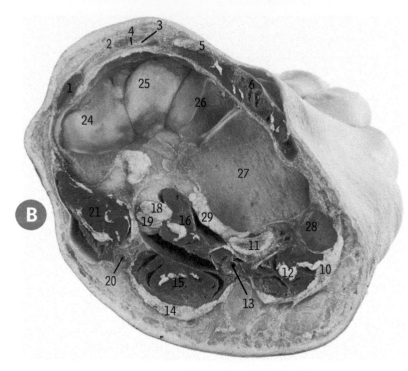

A Through the transverse tarsal joint, proximal to the navicular

B Through the cuneonavicular joint, distal to the navicular

Both sections are viewed from behind, looking from the heel toward the toes.

In A the section has passed through the talonavicular joint, so displaying the posterior (proximal) surface of the navicular (7). A small part of the cuboid (8) has been sliced off, leaving cartilage on the more lateral part of its posterior (calcanean) surface. The plantar aponeurosis (14) overlies flexor digitorum brevis (15), with abductor hallucis (21) on the medial side and abductor digiti minimi (12) laterally. Quadratus plantae (16) lies centrally, with the tendons of flexor hallucis longus (18) and flexor digitorum longus (19) more medially placed at this level.

In B at the level of the posterior (navicular) surfaces of the cuneiform bones, the tendon of flexor hallucis longus (18) is now passing deep to the digitorum tendon (19). The tendon of fibularis (*peroneus*) longus (11) is turning laterally under the cuboid (27), where a little more distally it will become covered by the long plantar ligament (29) (compare with the dissection on p. 99).

1 Tibialis anterior
2 Extensor hallucis longus
3 Dorsalis pedis artery
4 Deep fibular *(peroneal)* nerve
5 Extensor digitorum longus
6 Extensor digitorum brevis
7 Posterior articular surface of navicular (for talus)
8 Posterior articular surface of cuboid (for calcaneus)
9 Anterior tip of calcaneus
10 Fibularis *(peroneus)* brevis
11 Fibularis *(peroneus)* longus
12 Abductor digiti minimi
13 Lateral plantar nerve and vessels
14 Plantar aponeurosis
15 Flexor digitorum brevis
16 Quadratus plantae
17 Plantar calcaneocuboid (short plantar) ligament
18 Flexor hallucis longus
19 Flexor digitorum longus
20 Medial plantar nerve and vessels
21 Abductor hallucis
22 Tibialis posterior
23 Plantar calcaneonavicular (spring) ligament
24 Medial ⎫
25 Intermediate ⎬ cuneiform
26 Lateral ⎭
27 Cuboid
28 Tuberosity of fifth metatarsal
29 Long plantar ligament

Coronal sections of the right metatarsus

Both sections are viewed from behind, looking toward the toes. The metatarsals are numbered in Roman figures. On the dorsum the tendons of extensor digitorum longus to the appropriate toes are numbered L2–L5, and those of extensor digitorum brevis B2–B4 (recall that the brevis tendon to the great toe is named extensor hallucis brevis, 2). Similarly in the sole the flexor digitorum longus tendons are numbered L2–L5,

with the lumbrical muscles that arise from those tendons numbered U1–U4. The various interosseus muscles between and below the metatarsals have not been labeled.

In B note the sesamoid bones (18) under the head of the first metatarsal (I), with the tendon of flexor hallucis longus (8) between them.

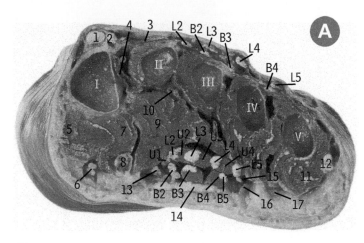

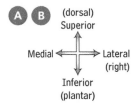

(dorsal)
Superior

Medial ⟷ Lateral
(right)

Inferior
(plantar)

1   Extensor hallucis longus
2   Extensor hallucis brevis
3   Arcuate artery
4   Deep plantar artery
5   Abductor hallucis
6   Proper plantar digital nerve of great toe
7   Flexor hallucis brevis
8   Flexor hallucis longus
9   Oblique head of adductor hallucis
10 Second plantar metatarsal artery
11 Flexor digiti minimi brevis
12 Abductor digiti minimi
13 Common plantar digital branches of medial plantar nerve
14 Plantar aponeurosis
15 Deep branch of lateral plantar nerve
16 Fourth common plantar digital nerve
17 Proper plantar digital nerve of fifth toe
18 Sesamoid bone
19 Transverse head of adductor hallucis

A Through the middle of the metatarsal shafts

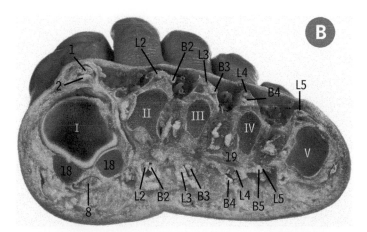

B Through the heads of the first and fifth metatarsals

Great toe *The dorsum, nail and sections of the great toe*

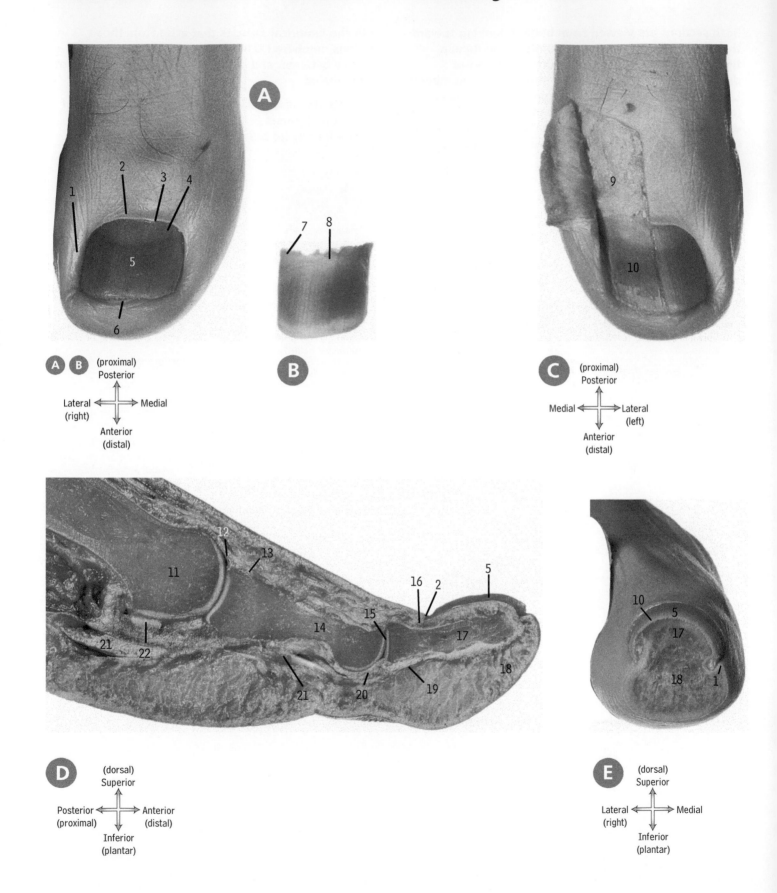

A

B

1
2
3
4
5
6
7
8

A **B** (proximal)
Posterior

Lateral ← → Medial
(right)

Anterior
(distal)

9
10

C (proximal)
Posterior

Medial ← → Lateral
(left)

Anterior
(distal)

11
12
13
14
15
16
2
5
17
18
19
20
21
21
22

D (dorsal)
Superior

Posterior ← → Anterior
(proximal)   (distal)

Inferior
(plantar)

10
5
17
18
1

E (dorsal)
Superior

Lateral ← → Medial
(right)

Inferior
(plantar)

A Dorsum of the right great toe

B Nail

C Nail bed of the left great toe

D Sagittal section of the right great toe, from the lateral side

E Coronal section of the distal phalanx of the right great toe

1 Nail wall
2 Nail fold
3 Eponychium
4 Lunule ⎤
5 Body ⎟
6 Free border ⎬ of nail
7 Occult border ⎟
8 Root ⎦
9 Germinal matrix ⎤ of nail bed
10 Sterile matrix ⎦
11 Head of first metatarsal
12 Capsule of metatarsophalangeal joint
13 Attachment of extensor hallucis brevis
14 Proximal phalanx
15 Capsule of interphalangeal joint
16 Attachment of extensor hallucis longus
17 Distal phalanx
18 Septa of pulp space
19 Attachment of flexor hallucis longus
20 Plantar ligament of interphalangeal joint
21 Flexor hallucis longus
22 Sesamoid bone

Imaging of the lower limb

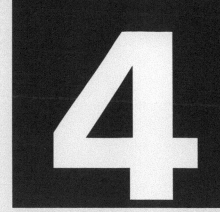

Lumbar spine *Plain radiographic and CT anatomy*

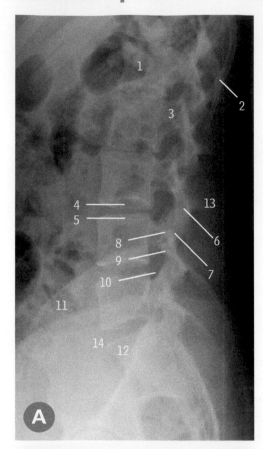

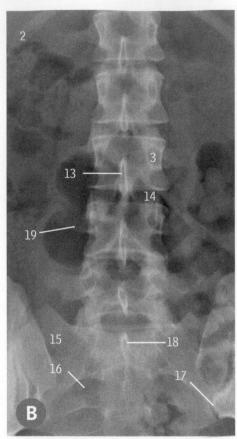

1 Body of L1 vertebra
2 12th rib
3 Pedicle of L2 vertebra
4 Inferior endplate of L3 vertebra
5 Superior endplate of L4 vertebra
6 Inferior articular process of L3 vertebra
7 Facet joint between L3 and L4 vertebrae
8 Superior articular process of L4 vertebra
9 Pars interarticularis
10 Neural foramen between L4 and L5 vertebrae
11 Wing of ilium
12 Body of S1 vertebra
13 Spinous process of L3 vertebra
14 Intervertebral disc space
15 Sacral ala
16 Second sacral neural foramen
17 Sacroiliac joint
18 Spinous process of S1
19 Transverse process of L4 vertebra
20 Sacral crest
21 Coccyx

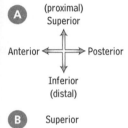

(proximal)
Superior

Anterior ⟷ Posterior

Inferior
(distal)

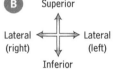

Superior

Lateral ⟷ Lateral
(right)   (left)

Inferior

Lateral (A) and anteroposterior (B) plain radiographs

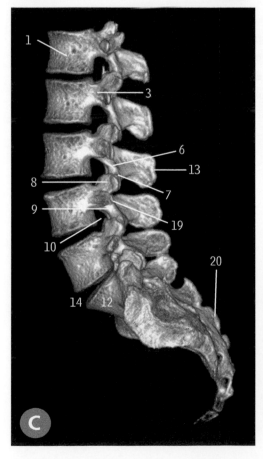

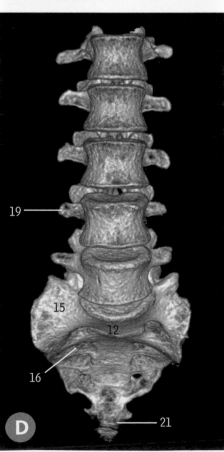

(proximal)
Superior

Anterior ⟷ Posterior

Inferior
(distal)

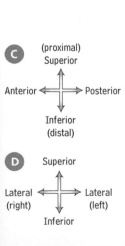

Superior

Lateral ⟷ Lateral
(right)   (left)

Inferior

Lateral (C) and anteroposterior (D) volume-rendered CT images

Lumbar spine *MRI anatomy—sagittal*

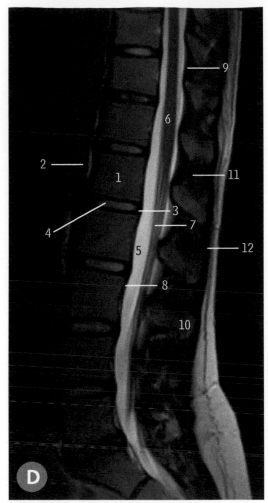

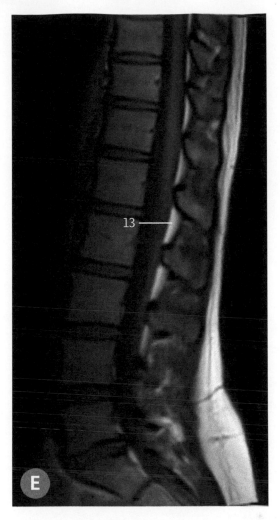

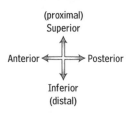

Sagittal T2-weighted (D) and T1-weighted (E) MR images

(proximal)
Superior

Anterior ⟸⟹ Posterior

Inferior
(distal)

1 Body of L1 vertebra	**10** Spinous process of L3
2 Anterior longitudinal ligament	vertebra
3 Annulus fibrosus of intervertebral disc	**11** Interspinous ligament
4 Nucleus pulposus	**12** Supraspinous ligament
5 Cerebrospinal fluid within dural sac	**13** Epidural fat
6 Conus medullaris of spinal cord	
7 Cauda equina	
8 Posterior longitudinal ligament	
9 Ligamentum flavum	

- The typical appearances of normal plain radiographic anatomy result from the superimposition of structures in both the lateral (**A**) and frontal (**B**) projections. The characteristic "owl's face" appearance of vertebrae on the frontal view (**B**) is accounted for by the "eyes" being formed by the pedicles (**B3**), and "beak" by the spinous process (**B13**); disruption of this normal appearance may be seen in disease, such as following tumour metastasis to the spine and in cases of trauma.

- (**C**) and (**D**) represent VRT ("Volume Rendered Technique") images acquired following computer-aided post-processing of Computed Tomographic (CT) data, a technique using X-rays. VRT images enable the selective visualization of bones and soft tissues which may subsequently be manipulated in three dimensions, an invaluable tool to the radiologist and surgeon. Virtual dissection, in which selected parts of anatomy are removed from images and which was used to obtain the images shown, can also be used to facilitate examination of inaccessible structures in three dimensions.

- Magnetic resonance imaging (MRI) provides detailed information on the soft tissues and bone marrow via the use of radio waves and strong magnetic fields, which may be manipulated in a variety of ways to selectively examine different tissue types. (**D**) demonstrates a "T2 weighted" image in which fluid, such as cerebrospinal fluid and that within the nucleus pulposus of intervertebral discs, appears bright ("high signal"). In "T1 weighted" images such as (**E**) fluid appears dark, while fat—such as that in the epidural space—is bright. Normal fat conversion of bone marrow occurs during ageing and is seen to manifest as relatively high signal within the vertebral bodies.

Lumbar spine *MRI anatomy—axial*

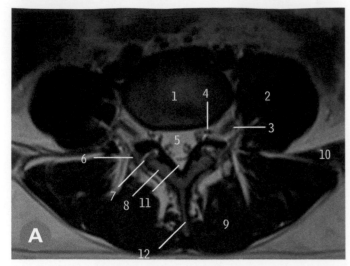
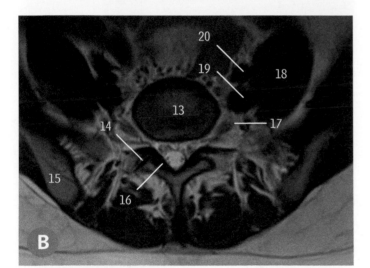

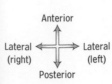

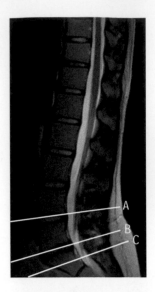

Axial T2-weighted MR images

Axial sections

1 Intervertebral disc between L4/L5
2 Psoas major
3 Exiting L4 nerve root
4 L5 nerve root within lateral recess
5 Thecal sac
6 Superior facet of L5 vertebra
7 Facet (zygapophyseal) joint of L4/L5
8 Inferior facet of L4 vertebra
9 Erector spinae
10 Quadratus lumborum
11 Epidural fat
12 Spinous process of L4 vertebra
13 Intervertebral disc between L5/S1
14 Facet (zygapophyseal) joint of L5/S1
15 Right wing of ilium
16 Ligamentum flavum
17 Exiting L5 nerve root
18 Psoas major
19 Left common iliac vein
20 Left common iliac artery
21 S1 vertebral body
22 Right sacral ala
23 Right sacroiliac joint
24 S1 nerve root

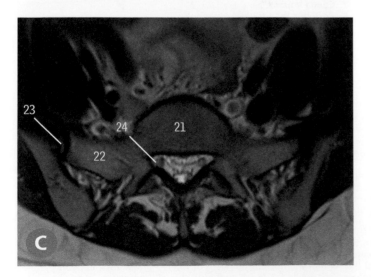

- Axial MR imaging of the spine, such as shown in images **A–C**, is invaluable in the assessment of intervertebral disc disease; herniation of disc material from the nucleus pulposus through the annulus fibrosus may compress the spinal cord (if occurring above the level of the cauda equina) or nerve roots either within the spinal canal or neural exit foramina.

Pelvis *Plain radiographic anatomy*

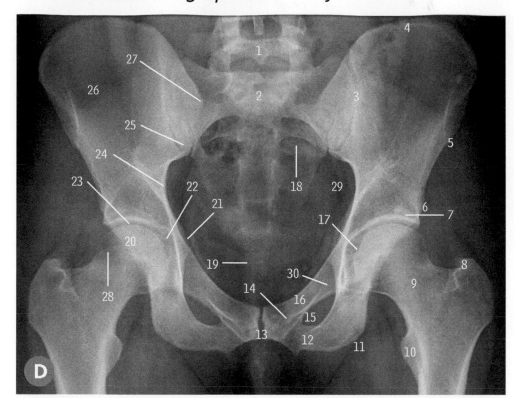
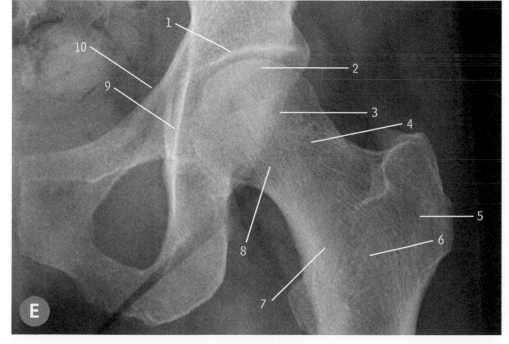

1 L5 vertebra
2 Sacrum
3 Sacroiliac joint
4 Iliac crest
5 Anterior superior } iliac spine
6 Anterior inferior
7 Roof of acetabulum
8 Greater trochanter of femur
9 Neck of femur
10 Lesser trochanter of femur
11 Ischial tuberosity
12 Inferior pubic ramus
13 Pubic symphysis
14 Pubic tubercle
15 Obturator foramen
16 Superior pubic ramus
17 Fovea capitis
18 Second sacral foramen
19 Coccyx
20 Head of femur
21 Ischial spine
22 Acetabular fossa
23 Hip joint space
24 Arcuate line
25 Posterior inferior iliac spine
26 Iliac wing
27 Posterior superior iliac spine
28 Epiphyseal line
29 Greater sciatic notch
30 Lesser sciatic notch (en face)

D Anteroposterior radiograph

1 Roof of acetabulum
2 Anterior wall of acetabulum
3 Posterior wall of acetabulum (en face)
4 Principle tensile group
5 Greater trochanter group
6 Secondary tensile group
7 Secondary } compressive group
8 Principle
9 Ilioischial line
10 Iliopectineal line

(proximal)
Superior

Medial ⟷ Lateral
(left)

Inferior
(distal)

E Left hip (magnified view)

• Among others, Julius Wolff (1836–1902), a German surgeon and anatomist, described the process by which organization of bone occurs in response to the stresses placed upon it as a result of gravity and dynamic forces—subsequently known as "Wolff's Law". This may be clearly seen in the organization and distribution of trabeculae (cancellous bone), a relatively lightweight form of bone that has a high surface area to mass ratio and that plays a key role in bone strength.

• Trabeculae can be seen to organize themselves in distinct patterns, which are well illustrated in the proximal femur (**E**). Classically, five groups of trabeculae (**E4-8**) can be reliably identified as a result of the compressive and tensile forces placed upon them. Long periods of inactivity (e.g. bed rest, spaceflight), in addition to age-related loss of bone mass (osteopaenia, osteoporosis), may result in weakening of trabeculae with resultant "insufficiency fractures". The femoral neck, as well as sacrum, pelvic bones and vertebral bodies, are commonly involved and such fractures are a major source of morbidity.

Pelvis *Male and female pelvis, sacrum*

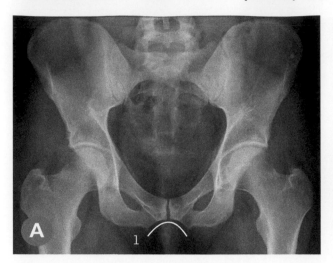

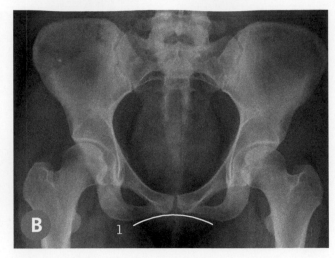

A Adult male pelvis radiograph

B Adult female pelvis radiograph

- Sex differences in the anatomy of the male and pelvis can be readily identified, although due to variation in the female pelvis (of which at least four types can be described—gynaecoid (50%), anthropoid (25%), android (20%) and platypelloid (5%)—not all may be seen in every individual.

- Classically, the following features may be seen:

  - Wider infrapubic angle (**A1**), >90 degrees in females, <90 degrees in males
  - Circular/oval pelvic inlet (females), heart-shaped (males)
  - Oval obturator foramen (females), rounded (males)
  - Wider sciatic notch (females)
  - Shorter, more triangular sacrum (females)
  - More anteriorly facing acetabulum (females)

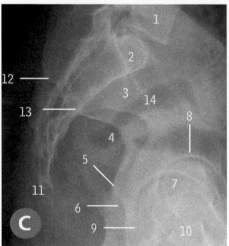

C Lateral radiograph of sacrum

(proximal)
Superior

Posterior ←→ Anterior

Inferior
(distal)

D Axial T1-weighted MR image of sacrum (S1/S2 level)

Anterior

Lateral (right) ←→ Lateral (left)

Posterior

1 Body of L5 vertebra	**9** Ramus of ischium	**17** Gluteus maximus
2 Sacrum	**10** Obturator foramen (en face)	**18** Right wing of ilium
3 Wing of ilium	**11** Coccyx	**19** Sacroiliac joint
4 Greater sciatic notch	**12** Posterior superior ⎫ iliac spine	**20** Sacral ala
5 Ischial spine	**13** Posterior inferior ⎭	**21** Second sacral foramen
6 Lesser sciatic notch	**14** Gas within rectum	**22** Multifidus/iliocostalis lumborum
7 Head of femur	**15** Gluteus minimus	**23** S2 nerve root
8 Roof of acetabulum	**16** Gluteus medius	**24** S1 nerve root

Pelvis *Developmental changes within the pelvis*

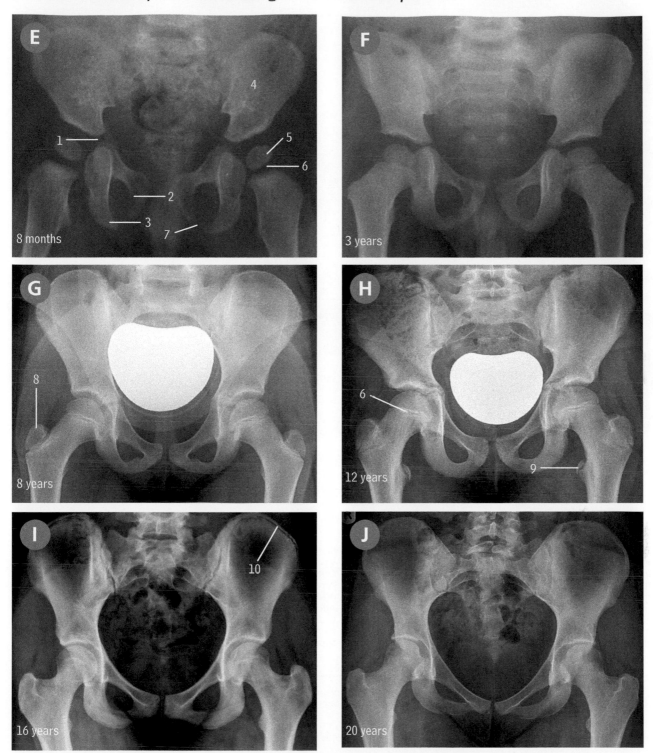

- Ossification of the pelvic bones progresses throughout infancy and childhood, with fusion not typically completing until 20–25 years of age. The pattern of ossification is predictable, depending on age, and may therefore be used to assess for delayed skeletal development.

- The triradiate cartilage (**E1**) represents the synchondrosis of the ilium, ischium and pubic bones and is an important landmark in the ultrasound assessment of infants for the presence of developmental dysplasia of the hip; in this condition, abnormal development of a shallow acetabulum occurs and predisposes the individual to subsequent subluxation and dislocation of the hip joint. If undetected, mobility may be affected in addition to the development of early-onset degenerative joint disease.

- Fusion of the iliac crest apophysis (*apophysis* = separate centre of ossification attached to a tendon or muscle, not forming part of a joint) is amongst the last to occur (**I10**), and can be seen to progress in a predictable pattern from laterally to medially.

1 Triradiate cartilage (synchondrosis)
2 Pubis
3 Ischium
4 Ilium
5 Femoral epiphysis
6 Proximal femoral physis (growth plate)
7 Ischiopubic synchondrosis
8 Greater ⎫ trochanter apophysis
9 Lesser ⎬
10 Iliac crest apophysis

Pelvis *MRI anatomy of the pelvis*

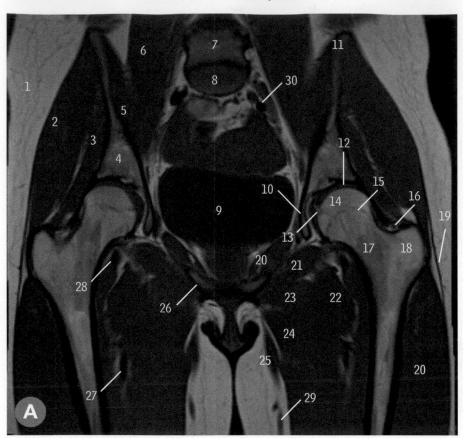

A

A Coronal T1-weighted MR image of the pelvis

Superior

Lateral ←——→ Lateral
(right)   (left)

Inferior

1 Subcutaneous fat	**10** Medial wall of acetabulum	**19** Iliotibial band	**28** Iliopsoas tendon
2 Gluteus medius	**11** Iliac crest	**20** Vastus lateralis	**29** Great saphenous vein
3 Gluteus minimus	**12** Articular cartilage	**21** Obturator externus	**30** External iliac artery and vein
4 Acetabulum	**13** Fovea capitis	**22** Pectineus	
5 Iliacus	**14** Femoral epiphysis	**23** Adductor minimus	
6 Psoas major	**15** Epiphyseal line	**24** Adductor brevis	
7 L5 vertebra	**16** Circumflex femoral vessels	**25** Gracilis	
8 S1 vertebra	**17** Neck of femur	**26** Pubic tubercle	
9 Urinary bladder	**18** Greater trochanter of femur	**27** Superficial femoral artery	

- Given the prevalence of chronic hip pain and the relative insensitivity of plain radiographs in the detection of pathology, MR imaging plays a critical role in assessment of the articular cartilage, periarticular bone and associated soft tissues.

- Fluoroscopically-guided injection of gadolinium-based contrast media into the hip joint space enables further evaluation, in particular of the articular cartilage and acetabular labrum. This is demonstrated in figures **B-E**, in which additional information on the structure of the various cartilaginous and ligamentous structures may be clearly seen.

Pelvis *MRI anatomy of the hip*

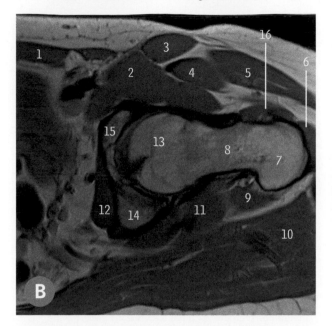

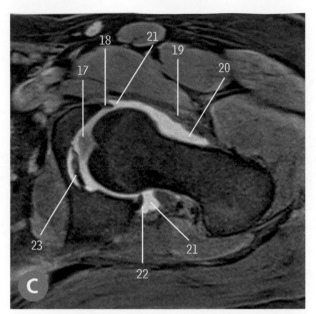

B C Axial T1 (C) and arthrogram (D) MR images of the left hip

Anterior

Medial ⟵⟶ Lateral (left)

Posterior

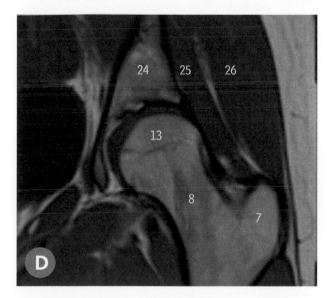

D E Coronal T1 (E) and arthrogram (F) MR images of the left hip

(proximal)
Superior

Medial ⟵⟶ Lateral (left)

Inferior
(distal)

1 Rectus abdominis	**9** Quadratus femoris	**17** Ligamentum teres (round ligament)	**23** Transverse acetabular ligament
2 Iliopsoas	**10** Gluteus maximus	**18** Anterior labrum	**24** Acetabulum
3 Sartorius	**11** Obturator externus	**19** Joint capsule	**25** Gluteus minimus
4 Rectus femoris	**12** Obturator internus	**20** Joint space (distended by contrast medium)	**26** Gluteus medius
5 Tensor fascia lata	**13** Head of femur	**21** Perilabral sulcus	**27** Superior labrum
6 Gluteus medius	**14** Ischium	**22** Posterior labrum	**28** Superior perilabral recess
7 Greater trochanter of femur	**15** Pubis		**29** Zona orbicularis
8 Neck of femur	**16** Vastus lateralis		

Arterial anatomy *MRA angiographic anatomy of the pelvis and leg*

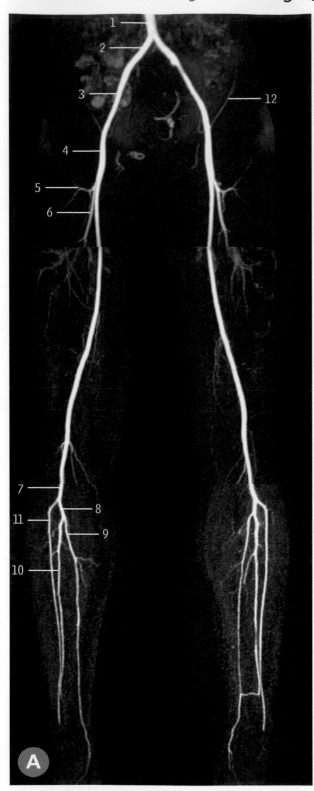

- Recent years have seen a paradigm shift in techniques used in the assessment of the vasculature. Previously, digital subtraction angiography (DSA) was widely used in a diagnostic role, requiring puncture of a vessel, placement of an indwelling catheter, and injection of radiopaque contrast media (**B**).

- Notwithstanding the radiation burden to the patient, the use of such a technique also involved the attendant risks and potential complications of vascular puncture as well as adverse reactions to relatively high doses of iodine-based contrast media.

- Although still used in a therapeutic role (e.g. angioplasty), DSA has essentially been replaced by noninvasive techniques in the investigation of patients for potential vascular disease.

- Computed tomographic angiography (CTA) is a minimally invasive technique involving the use of CT imaging in conjunction with iodine-based contrast media, injected via a small cannula typically sited within a peripheral vein. This is in contrast to DSA, in which a specialized catheter requires placement either close to or within the vessel of interest itself and which uses significantly higher volumes of contrast media.

- Evaluation of the data acquired allows assessment for the development of significant atherosclerotic disease, in particular the presence of stenoses (narrowings) of vessels that may require subsequent treatment, as well as assessment for vascular integrity in the context of trauma and haemorrhage.

- Volume rendered technique (VRT) images may also be produced from datasets, thereby providing three dimensional information not available using DSA (**C, D**). Figure (**C**) clearly shows the relationship of the femoral artery to the femoral head posteriorly; this is of clinical use in the context of the acute management of major trauma to the leg, in which direct compression of the artery against the femoral head posteriorly may be employed to temporarily reduce or stop haemorrhage prior to definitive management.

- Magnetic resonance angiography (MRA) is a further technique which employs gadolinium-based contrast media and avoids the use of ionizing radiation (**A**). In certain circumstances, using special techniques, the use of contrast media may be avoided entirely via the evaluation of the physical properties of flowing blood in a strong magnetic field. This is less commonly used in the evaluation of the vasculature of the lower limb, however, and is more prone to image artefact, which may make interpretation challenging.

- Maximum intensity projection (MIP) images, such as in (**A**), are employed in both CTA and MRA. In this technique, only the points of highest signal (MR) or radiodensity (CT) are displayed, thereby allowing the rapid evaluation of a large body area but without the three dimensional information provided by VRT images.

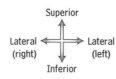

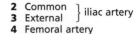

Superior

Lateral (right) ⟷ Lateral (left)

Inferior

(A) **Coronal T1-weighted Maximum Intensity Projection (MIP) MR angiogram of the legs**

1 Abdominal aorta
2 Common } iliac artery
3 External
4 Femoral artery
5 Lateral circumflex femoral artery
6 Profunda femoris
7 Popliteal artery
8 Tibiofibular (tibioperoneal) trunk
9 Posterior } tibial artery
10 Anterior
11 Fibular (peroneal) artery
12 Superficial circumflex iliac artery

Arterial anatomy *Arterial anatomy of the hip*

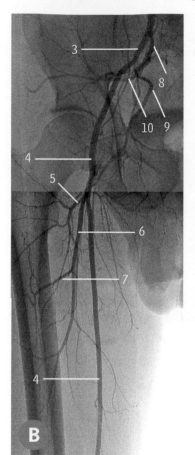

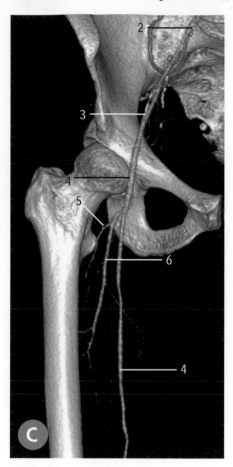

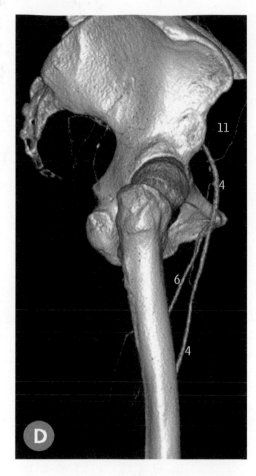

B Anteroposterior digital subtraction angiogram of the right hip

C Anteroposterior (C) and lateral (D) volume-
D rendered CT angiogram images of the right hip

E Lateral T1-weighted Maximum Intensity Projection (MIP) MR angiogram of the pelvis

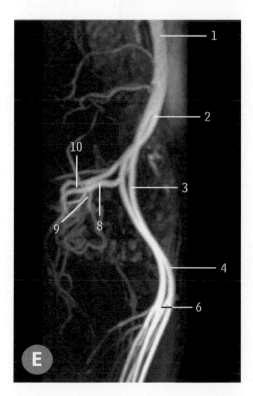

1 Abdominal aorta
2 Common } iliac artery
3 External }
4 Femoral artery
5 Lateral circumflex femoral artery
6 Profunda femoris
7 Perforating artery
8 Internal iliac artery
9 Anterior } division of internal iliac artery
10 Posterior }
11 Superficial epigastric artery

B **C**   Superior
Lateral ⟷ Medial
(right)
Inferior

D **E**   Superior
Posterior ⟷ Anterior
Inferior

Thigh *MRI anatomy of the thigh—coronal*

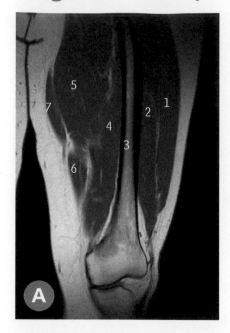
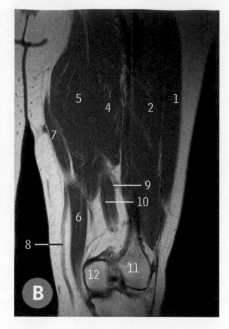
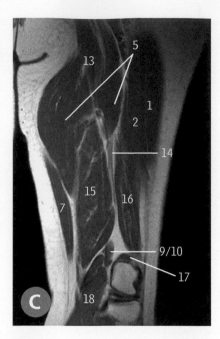

Ⓐ Ⓑ Ⓒ **Coronal T1-weighted MR images of the left thigh**

(proximal)
Superior

Medial ⟷ Lateral
(left)

Inferior
(distal)

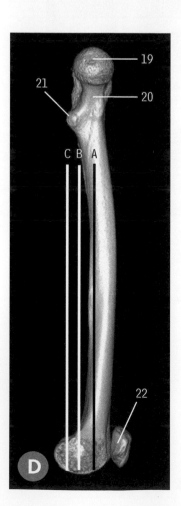

Ⓓ **Volume-rendered CT image of the left leg, medial view**

1 Vastus lateralis	**12** Medial condyle of femur
2 Vastus intermedius	**13** Semitendinosus
3 Shaft of femur	**14** Sciatic nerve
4 Vastus medialis	**15** Semimembranosus
5 Adductor magnus	**16** Biceps femoris
6 Sartorius	**17** Lateral } head of gastrocnemius
7 Gracilis	**18** Medial
8 Great saphenous vein	**19** Head of femur
9 Femoral artery	**20** Neck of femur
10 Femoral vein	**21** Lesser trochanter of femur
11 Lateral condyle of femur	**22** Patella

Thigh *MRI anatomy of the thigh—axial*

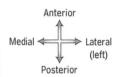

Axial T1-weighted MR images of the left thigh

Anterior

Medial ⟷ Lateral (left)

Posterior

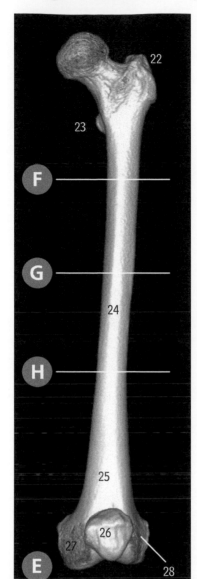

E **Volume-rendered CT image of the left femur, anterior view**

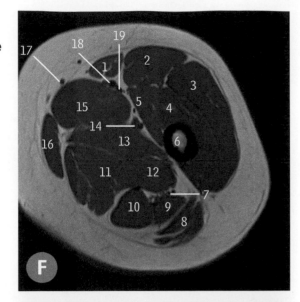

F

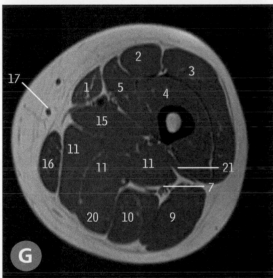

G

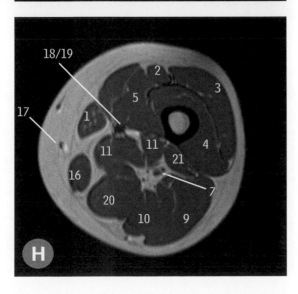

H

1	Sartorius	**15**	Adductor longus
2	Rectus femoris	**16**	Gracilis
3	Vastus lateralis	**17**	Great saphenous vein
4	Vastus intermedius	**18**	Femoral artery
5	Vastus medialis	**19**	Femoral vein
6	Femur	**20**	Semimembranosus
7	Sciatic nerve	**21**	Biceps femoris (short head)
8	Gluteus maximus	**22**	Greater ⎫ trochanter of femur
9	Biceps femoris (long head)	**23**	Lesser ⎭
10	Semitendinosus	**24**	Femoral shaft (diaphysis)
11	Adductor magnus	**25**	Distal metaphysis
12	Adductor minimus	**26**	Patella
13	Adductor brevis	**27**	Medial ⎫ condyle of femur
14	Profunda femoris and deep femoral vein	**28**	Lateral ⎭

Knee *Plain radiographic anatomy*

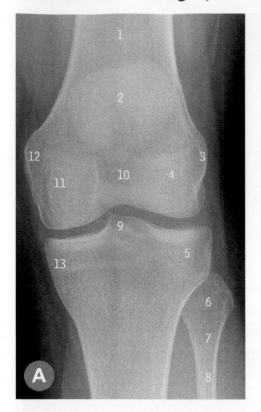

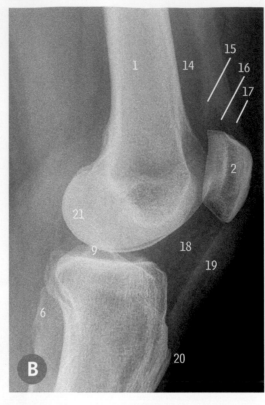

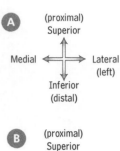

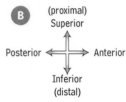

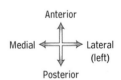

Ⓐ Ⓑ Anteroposterior (A) and lateral (B) radiographs of the left knee

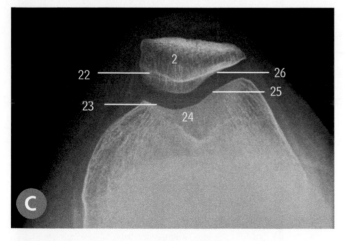

1 Femur	**19** Patellar tendon
2 Patella	**20** Tibial tuberosity
3 Lateral epicondyle of femur	**21** Femoral condyles (*en face*)
4 Lateral condyle of femur	**22** Medial patellar facet
5 Lateral condyle of tibia	**23** Medial trochlear facet
6 Head of fibula	**24** Trochlea
7 Neck of fibula	**25** Lateral trochlear facet
8 Proximal shaft of fibula	**26** Lateral patellar facet
9 Intercondylar eminence	
10 Intercondylar fossa	
11 Medial condyle of femur	
12 Medial epicondyle of femur	
13 Medial condyle of tibia	
14 Prefemoral fat pad	
15 Suprapatellar bursa	
16 Quadriceps fat pad	
17 Quadriceps tendon	
18 Infrapatellar fat pad (of Hoffa)	

Ⓒ "Skyline" or "sunrise" view of the left patellofemoral joint

- The "skyline" or "sunrise" view of the patellofemoral joint as shown in (C) is used most often to evaluate for the development of degenerative joint disease, assessment for possible fractures and for the evaluation of femoral trochlear dysplasia in which an abnormally shallow or flattened trochlear surface predisposes individuals to dislocation of the patella.

- As seen in (C), the normal lateral trochlear facet is steeper and longer than that on the medial side; despite this, lateral dislocation of the patella is far more common than medial dislocation, in part due to the biomechanic forces at the time of injury. Disruption of the medial patellofemoral ligaments frequently occurs, resulting in subsequent instability that may necessitate surgical intervention.

- As demonstrated in (D3), traumatic injury to the knee, in particular the head and neck of the fibula, may also result in injury to the common fibular nerve as it passes lateral to the bone where it is vulnerable to crushing forces. As a result, disabling weakness to the muscles of the calf may occur, resulting in foot drop and paraesthesia (skin sensory changes).

Knee *MRI anatomy of the knee—sagittal*

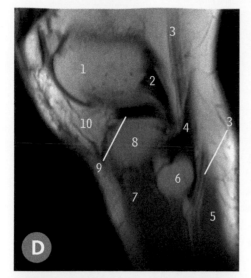

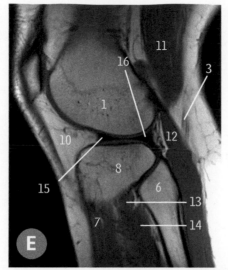

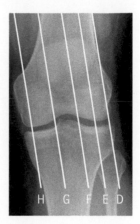

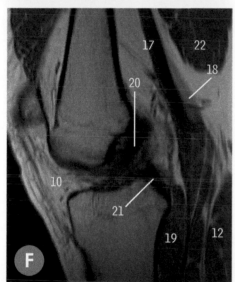

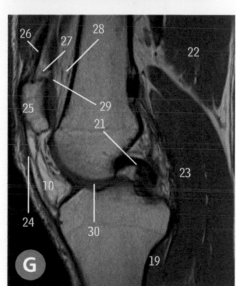

Superior
(proximal)

Anterior ⟷ Posterior

Inferior
(distal)

D-H

Sagittal T1-weighted MR images of the left knee

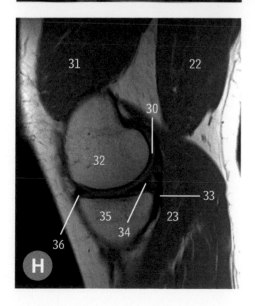

1 Lateral condyle of femur	**19** Popliteus
2 Fibular collateral ligament	**20** Anterior cruciate ligament
3 Common fibular (peroneal) nerve	**21** Posterior cruciate ligament
4 Biceps femoris tendon	**22** Semimembranosus
5 Soleus	**23** Medial head of gastrocnemius
6 Head of fibula	**24** Patella tendon
7 Tibialis anterior	**25** Patella
8 Lateral condyle of tibia	**26** Quadriceps tendon
9 Lateral meniscus	**27** Quadriceps fat pad
10 Infrapatellar fat pad (of Hoffa)	**28** Prefemoral fat pad
11 Biceps femoris	**29** Suprapatellar bursa
12 Lateral head of gastrocnemius	**30** Femoral articular cartilage
13 Extensor digitorum longus	**31** Vastus medialis
14 Tibialis posterior	**32** Medial condyle of femur
15 Anterior ⎫ head of lateral meniscus	**33** Oblique popliteal ligament/joint capsule
16 Posterior ⎭	**34** Posterior horn of medial meniscus
17 Popliteal artery and vein	**35** Medial condyle of tibia
18 Tibial nerve	**36** Anterior horn of medial meniscus

Knee *MRI anatomy of the knee—coronal and axial*

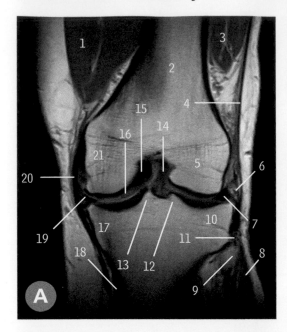
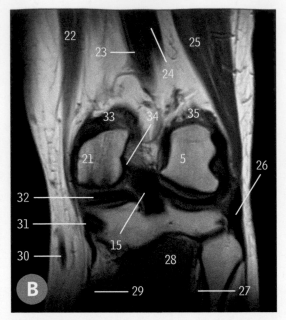
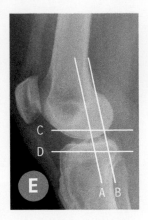

Ⓐ Ⓑ Coronal T1-weighted MR images of the left knee

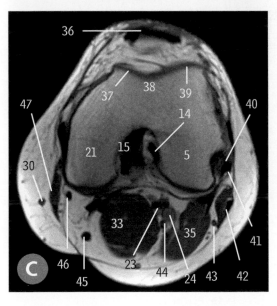
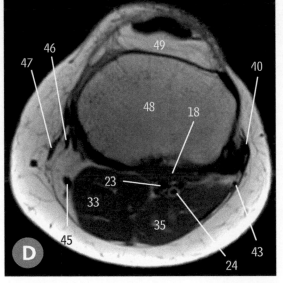

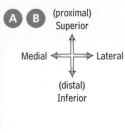

Ⓐ Ⓑ (proximal) Superior

Medial ⟷ Lateral

(distal) Inferior

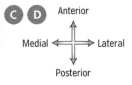

Ⓒ Ⓓ Anterior

Medial ⟷ Lateral

Posterior

Ⓒ Ⓓ Axial T1-weighted MR images of the left knee

1 Vastus medialis
2 Femur
3 Vastus lateralis
4 Iliotibial tract
5 Lateral condyle of femur
6 Lateral inferior genicular artery
7 Lateral meniscus
8 Fibularis (peroneus) longus
9 Head of fibula
10 Lateral condyle of tibia
11 Anterior ligament of the fibular head
12 Lateral } intercondylar tubercle
13 Medial

14 Anterior cruciate ligament
15 Posterior cruciate ligament
16 Articular cartilage
17 Medial condyle of tibia
18 Popliteus
19 Medial meniscus
20 Medial collateral ligament
21 Medial condyle of femur
22 Sartorius
23 Popliteal vein
24 Popliteal artery
25 Biceps femoris, short head
26 Biceps femoris tendon
27 Soleus
28 Popliteus

29 Medial head of gastrocnemius
30 Great saphenous vein
31 Semimembranosus tendon
32 Posterior horn of medial meniscus
33 Medial head of gastrocnemius
34 Posterior meniscofemoral ligament (of Wrisberg)
35 Lateral head of gastrocnemius
36 Patellar ligament
37 Medial trochlear facet
38 Trochlea

39 Lateral trochlear facet
40 Fibular (lateral) collateral ligament
41 Joint capsule
42 Biceps muscle and tendon
43 Common fibular (peroneal) nerve
44 Tibial nerve
45 Semitendinosus tendon
46 Gracilis tendon
47 Sartorius
48 Tibia
49 Infrapatellar fat pad (of Hoffa)

Knee *Arterial anatomy of the knee—DSA, CT*

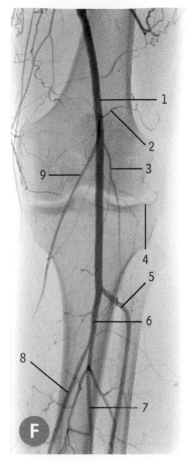

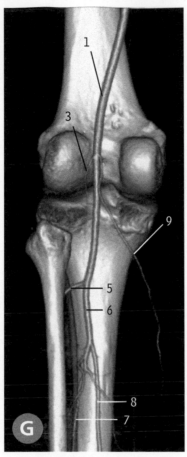

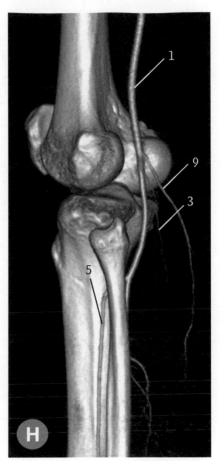

F Anteroposterior digital subtraction angiogram of the left knee

G **H** Volume-rendered CT image of the left knee, posterior view (G), lateral view (H)

1 Popliteal artery
2 Lateral superior genicular artery
3 Lateral sural artery
4 Lateral inferior genicular artery
5 Anterior tibial artery
6 Tibiofibular (tibioperoneal) trunk
7 Fibular (peroneal) artery
8 Posterior tibial artery
9 Medial sural artery

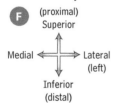

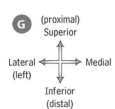

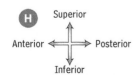

- In general, in clinical practice the term *peroneal* (Greek origin) is favoured over the term *fibular* (Latin orig.) as preferred by anatomists, when describing the muscles, nerves and vessels of the lower limb. Throughout this chapter, both may be considered synonymously but with the latter favoured.

- Furthermore, although not routinely recognized by anatomists, in clinical practice—and in particular in the context of interventional radiology and vascular surgery—the term **tibioperoneal** (tibiofibular) **trunk** (**F, G 6**) is used to describe the short section of artery between the origin of the anterior tibial and posterior tibial/fibular (peroneal) arteries, frequently affected by atherosclerotic disease along with its neighbouring vessels.

- Although there is relatively little variation in iliac or femoral arterial anatomy, considerable variation exists in the anatomy of the distal popliteal artery, in particular, the level and pattern of origins of the fibular (peroneal), anterior tibial and posterior tibial arteries.

- Figures **F, G** and **H** demonstrate the commonest pattern, seen in up to 90% of individuals, in which the popliteal artery divides at the inferior border of the popliteal muscle, continuing as the **tibioperoneal** trunk which subsequently gives rise to the anterior tibial and fibular (peroneal) arteries.

- In the remaining 10%, at least nine variant patterns are recognized, of varying frequency; although the anterior tibial artery invariably represents the first division, this, in addition to the origin of the posterior tibial artery, may occur above the level of the knee joint. The tibial artery may also be hypoplastic (poorly developed) or absent completely, the blood supply to the foot being provided exclusively by the anterior tibial and fibular (peroneal) arteries and their branches.

- Such variation is not simply of academic interest: failure to recognize variant anatomy may have significant consequences when surgical or interventional procedures are planned that in extreme cases may impact on limb salvage.

Knee *Arterial anatomy of the knee—CT, MRI*

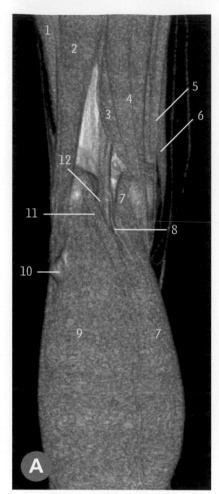

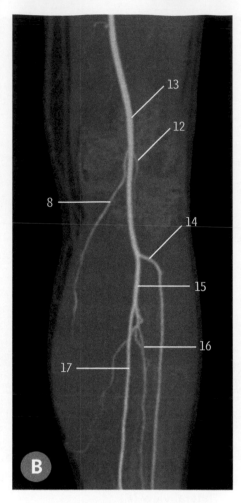

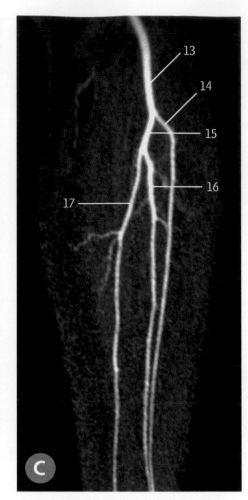

A Volume-rendered CT image of the left knee, posterior view of popliteal fossa

B Coronal Maximum Intensity Projection (MIP) CT angiogram of the left knee, viewed from anteriorly

C Coronal Maximum Intensity Projection (MIP) MR angiogram of the left knee, viewed from anteriorly

1 Vastus lateralis
2 Biceps femoris
3 Semimembranosus
4 Semitendinosus
5 Gracilis
6 Sartorius
7 Medial head of gastrocnemius
8 Medial sural artery
9 Lateral head of gastrocnemius
10 Head of fibula
11 Plantaris
12 Lateral sural artery
13 Popliteal artery
14 Anterior tibial artery
15 Tibiofibular (tibioperoneal) trunk
16 Fibular (peroneal) artery
17 Posterior tibial artery

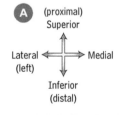

A (proximal)
Superior

Lateral ⟵⟶ Medial
(left)

Inferior
(distal)

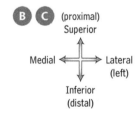

B C (proximal)
Superior

Medial ⟵⟶ Lateral
(left)

Inferior
(distal)

- Figure **A**, in addition to figures **G** and **H** on page 17, elegantly show the vulnerability of the popliteal artery to injury, in particular following traumatic posterior dislocation in which the artery may be compressed between the dislocated distal femur and posterior soft tissues; this may result in an acute and complete interruption to the lower leg blood supply requiring emergency intervention. A CT scan performed as part of trauma imaging protocols allows the rapid assessment of the lower limb vasculature in such cases.

- Certain individuals, due to variant anatomy, experience intermittent compression of the popliteal artery by the adjacent musculotendinous structures (most often the medial head of gastrocnemius) against the medial condyle of the femur. Magnetic resonance angiography (**C**) of the lower limbs allows the evaluation of the vasculature in such cases and enables the radiologist to determine the precise relationships of the popliteal vasculature and adjacent muscles due to much greater soft tissue contrast when compared with CT.

Lower leg *MRI anatomy of the lower leg—coronal*

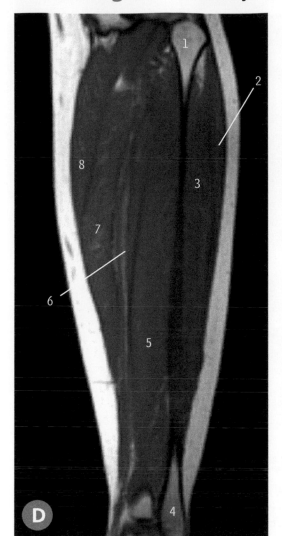

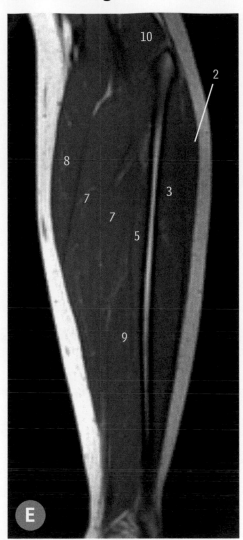

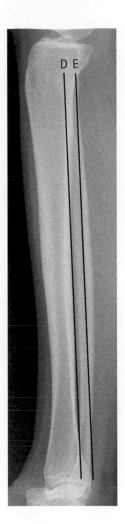

D E **Coronal T1-weighted MR images of the left calf**

D E (proximal)
Superior

Medial ⟷ Lateral
(left)

Inferior
(distal)

1 Head of fibula
2 Fibularis (peroneus) longus
3 Fibularis (peroneus) brevis
4 Lateral malleolus of fibula
5 Tibialis posterior
6 Tibial artery and nerve
7 Soleus
8 Medial head of gastrocnemius
9 Flexor hallucis longus
10 Lateral head of gastrocnemius

Lower leg *MRI anatomy of the lower leg—axial*

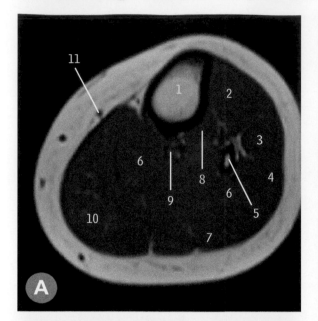

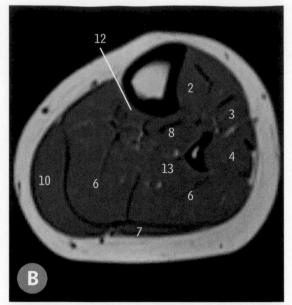

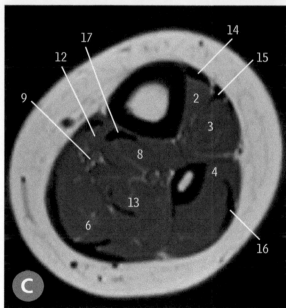

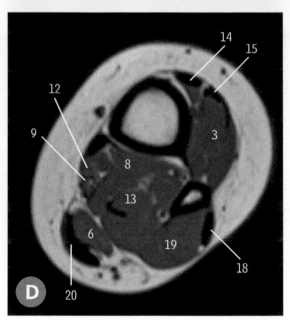

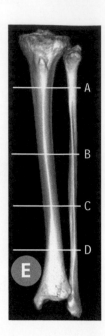

A-**D** Axial T1-weighted MR images of the left calf

Anterior
↑
Medial ←——→ Lateral
(left)
↓
Posterior

1 Tibia
2 Tibialis anterior
3 Extensor hallucis longus and extensor digitorum longus
4 Fibularis (peroneus) longus and brevis
5 Fibula
6 Soleus
7 Lateral head of gastrocnemius
8 Tibialis posterior
9 Posterior tibial artery and tibial nerve
10 Medial head of gastrocnemius

11 Great saphenous vein
12 Flexor digitorum longus
13 Flexor hallucis longus
14 Tibialis anterior tendon
15 Extensor digitorum longus tendon
16 Fibularis (peroneus) longus and brevis tendon
17 Tibialis posterior tendon
18 Fibularis (peroneus) longus tendon
19 Fibularis (peroneus) brevis
20 Tendo calcaneus (Achilles tendon)

Ankle *Plain radiographic anatomy*

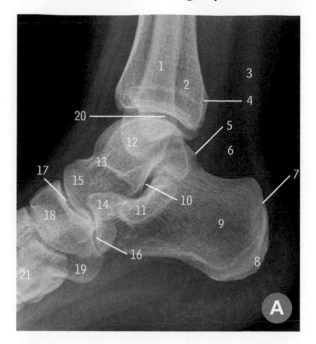

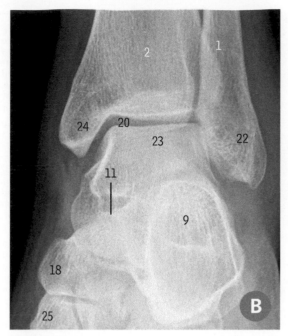

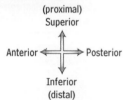

A Lateral radiograph of the left ankle

(proximal)
Superior

Anterior ⟷ Posterior

Inferior
(distal)

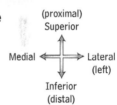

B Anteroposterior radiograph of the left ankle

(proximal)
Superior

Medial ⟷ Lateral
(left)

Inferior
(distal)

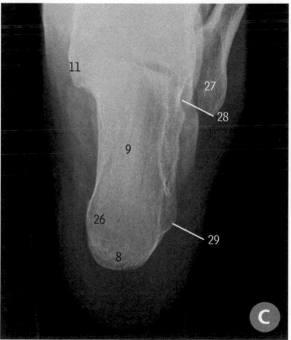

C Axial radiograph of the left calcaneus

Anterior

Medial ⟷ Lateral
(left)

Posterior

1 Fibula
2 Tibia
3 Tendo calcaneus (Achilles tendon)
4 Posterior process of tibia
5 Posterior process of talus
6 Pre-Achilles fat pad (of Kager)
7 Posterior surface of calcaneus
8 Calcaneal tuberosity
9 Calcaneus
10 Subtalar (talocalcaneal) joint
11 Sustentaculum tali
12 Body } of talus
13 Neck
14 Anterior process of calcaneus
15 Head of talus
16 Calcaneocuboid joint
17 Talonavicular joint
18 Navicular
19 Cuboid
20 Tibiotalar joint
21 Cuneiform bones (en face)
22 Lateral malleolus of fibula
23 Talar dome
24 Medial malleolus of fibula
25 Medial cuneiform
26 Medial process of calcaneus
27 Base of fifth metatarsal
28 Groove for fibularis (peroneus) longus
29 Lateral process of calcaneus

Ankle *MRI anatomy of the ankle—sagittal*

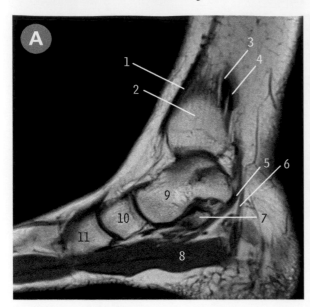

- The *subtalar joint* is a complex joint of the hindfoot comprised of the *talocalcaneal joint* posteriorly between the posterior talar and calcaneal facets (**B16**) and *talocalcaneonavicular joint* more anteriorly; the latter is formed by congruent articulations between the head of the talus, anterior and middle articular facets of the calcaneus and posterior articular facet of the navicular. Functionally, the subtalar joint plays a key role in imparting stability to the midfoot and hindfoot and allows pronation and supination, of importance when walking on uneven surfaces and during running.

- The *sinus tarsi* (**B17**) is a fat-filled space between the talus and calcaneus; its boundary is formed by the neck of the talus medially, calcaneus inferiorly and extensor retinaculum laterally. Contained within the sinus are the cervical and interosseous talocalcaneal ligaments, in addition to extensive nerve endings. Injury to the ligaments or haemorrhage within the sinus following trauma may result in instability, inflammation of synovium and the formation of scar tissue. The resultant symptoms of pain and persistent hindfoot instability are known as *sinus tarsi syndrome* and are particularly recognized in overweight individuals, those with 'flat feet' and in those with occupations predisposing them to repetitive injury.

- The *tarsal tunnel* (**E18**) lies medially within the ankle, has a boundary formed by the flexor retinaculum (laciniate ligament), talus and calcaneus and contains the posterior tibial neuromuscular bundle, tibialis posterior tendon and tendons of flexor digitorum longus and flexor hallucis longus. Swelling within the tunnel or compression from external sources—for example, due to the presence of accessory muscles (e.g. Flexor digitorum accessorius longus), tumours or scar tissue—may result in compression of the posterior tibial nerve or its branches. Those affected report pain and abnormal sensation along the medial foot and hallux, symptoms that are exacerbated by exercise. Surgical release by transecting the flexor retinaculum may be required to relieve symptoms.

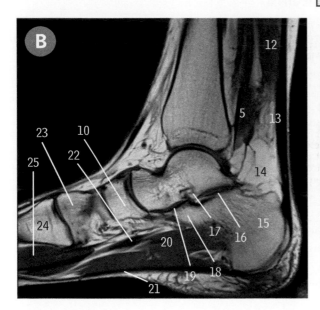

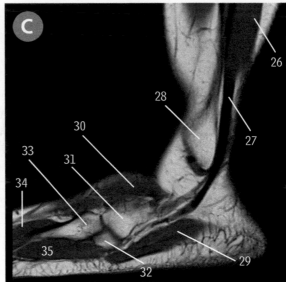

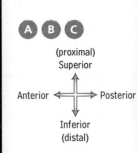

(proximal)
Superior

Anterior ⟷ Posterior

Inferior
(distal)

Ⓐ Ⓑ Ⓒ Sagittal T1-weighted MR images of the left ankle

1 Great saphenous vein	**14** Pre-Achilles fat pad (of Kager)	**26** Fibularis (peroneus) brevis
2 Tibia	**15** Calcaneus	**27** Fibularis (peroneus) longus
3 Tibialis posterior tendon	**16** Posterior talocalcaneal facet	tendon
4 Flexor digitorum longus tendon	**17** Sinus tarsi	**28** Lateral malleolus of fibula
5 Flexor hallucis longus tendon	**18** Anterior process of calcaneus	**29** Abductor digiti minimi
6 Tibial nerve	**19** Middle talocalcaneal joint	**30** Extensor digitorum brevis
7 Sustentaculum tali	**20** Quadratus plantae	and extensor hallucis brevis
8 Flexor digitorum brevis	**21** Plantar aponeurosis	**31** Cuboid
9 Talus	**22** Flexor digitorum longus and	**32** Base of fifth metatarsal
10 Navicular	flexor hallucis longus tendons	**33** Fourth metatarsal
11 Medial cuneiform	**23** Intermediate cuneiform	**34** Dorsal interosseous
12 Soleus	**24** Second metatarsal	**35** Flexor digiti minimi
13 Tendo calcaneus (Achilles tendon)	**25** Adductor hallucis	

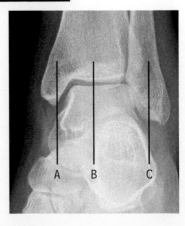

Ankle *MRI anatomy of the ankle—axial*

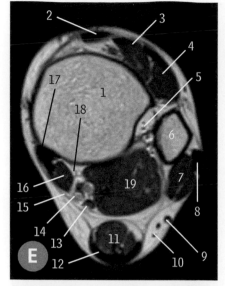

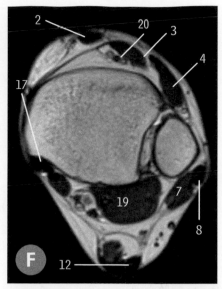

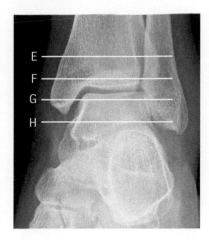

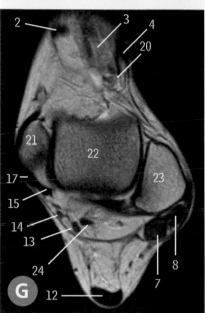

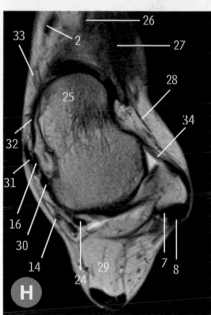

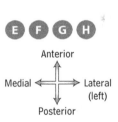

Anterior

Medial ⟷ Lateral
(left)

Posterior

E-H Axial T1-weighted MR images of the left ankle

1 Tibia
2 Tibialis anterior tendon
3 Extensor hallucis longus muscle and tendon
4 Extensor digitorum longus muscle and tendon
5 Fibular (peroneal) artery and vein
6 Fibula
7 Fibularis (peroneus) brevis
8 Fibularis (peroneus) longus tendon
9 Lesser (small) saphenous vein
10 Sural nerve
11 Soleus
12 Tendo calcaneus (Achilles tendon)
13 Tibial nerve
14 Posterior tibial artery and vein
15 Flexor retinaculum
16 Flexor digitorum longus muscle and tendon
17 Tibialis posterior tendon
18 Tarsal tunnel
19 Flexor hallucis longus muscle and tendon
20 Anterior tibial artery and deep fibular (peroneal) nerve
21 Medial malleolus of tibia
22 Talus
23 Lateral malleolus of tibia
24 Flexor hallucis longus tendon
25 Head of talus
26 Extensor hallucis longus tendon
27 Extensor digitorum brevis
28 Extensor retinaculum
29 Pre-Achilles fat pad (of Kager)
30 Flexor digitorum longus tendon
31 Deltoid ligament (tibiocalcaneal)
32 Deltoid ligament (tibionavicular)
33 Great saphenous vein
34 Anterior talofibular ligament

Ankle *MRI anatomy of the ankle—coronal and ultrasound anatomy*

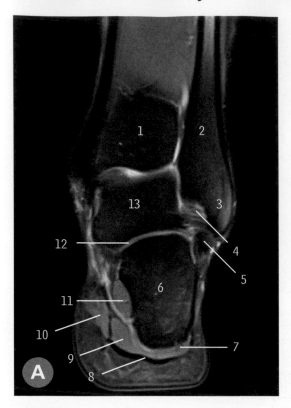

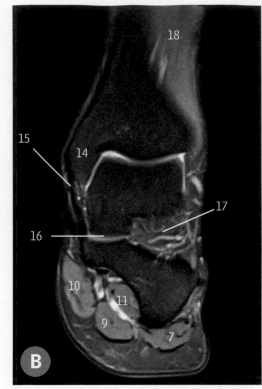

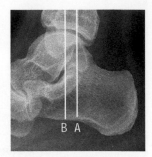

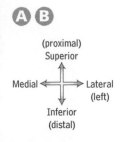

(proximal)
Superior

Medial ⟷ Lateral
(left)

Inferior
(distal)

Ⓐ Ⓑ **Coronal proton-density fat saturated MR images of the left ankle**

1	Tibia	**13**	Talus
2	Fibula	**14**	Medial malleolus of tibia
3	Lateral malleolus of fibula	**15**	Deltoid (medial collateral)
4	Posterior talofibular ligament		ligament
5	Fibularis (peroneus) longus	**16**	Middle talar facet
	and brevis tendons	**17**	Sinus tarsi
6	Calcaneus	**18**	Extensor digitorum longus
7	Abductor digiti minimi		and fibularis (peroneus) tertius
8	Plantar aponeurosis	**19**	Tendo calcaneus (Achilles
9	Flexor digitorum brevis		tendon)
10	Abductor hallucis	**20**	Pre-Achilles fat pad (of Kager)
11	Quadratus plantae	**21**	Skin surface
12	Posterior talocalcaneal facet		

- Ultrasound evaluation of musculotendinous structures is now standard in the evaluation of those with musculoskeletal disease, due to its ease of availability, lack of expense, high resolution and the ability to image tendons and ligaments during active and passive movement.

- Figures C and D demonstrate high resolution ultrasound images of the Achilles tendon (C19) in longitudinal and axial (transverse) orientations respectively. The ordered pattern of parallel collagen fibres are clearly seen as they course toward their insertion on the calcaneus (A6).

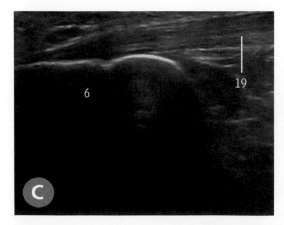

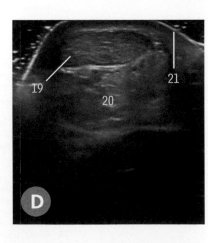

Ⓒ **Longitudinal ultrasound image of the left Achilles tendon and calcaneus**

Posterior

Distal ⟷ Proximal

Anterior

Ⓓ **Axial ultrasound image of the left Achilles tendon**

Posterior

Medial ⟷ Lateral
(left)

Anterior

Foot *Plain radiographic anatomy*

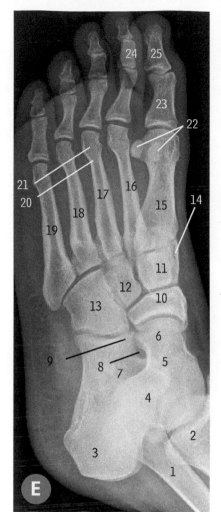

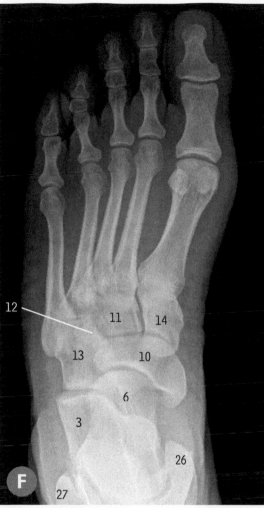

1 Fibula
2 Tibia
3 Calcaneus
4 Body ⎫
5 Neck ⎬ of talus
6 Head ⎭
7 Neck of calcaneus
8 Sinus tarsi
9 Anterior process of calcaneus
10 Navicular
11 Intermediate cuneiform
12 Lateral cuneiform
13 Cuboid
14 Medial cuneiform
15 First ⎫
16 Second │
17 Third ⎬ metatarsal
18 Fourth │
19 Fifth ⎭
20 Neck ⎫ of third metatarsal
21 Head ⎭
22 Sesamoid bones
23 Proximal ⎫
24 Middle ⎬ phalanx
25 Distal ⎭
26 Medial ⎫ malleolus of tibia
27 Lateral ⎭
28 Intermetatarsal ligaments
29 Dorsal ligaments
30 Dorsal intertarsal ligaments
31 Lisfranc joint complex
32 Lisfranc joint
33 Dorsal Lisfranc ligament

E F

Oblique (E) and dorsoplantar (F) radiographs of the left foot

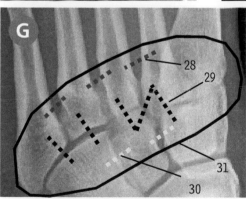

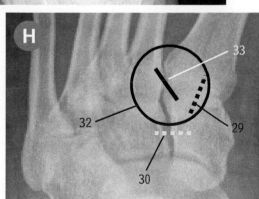

G H

Magnified oblique (G) and dorsoplantar (H) radiographs of the left tarsometatarsal joints

- *Jacques Lisfranc de St. Martin (1790–1847)* was a French surgeon and gynaecologist who served as a field surgeon in Napoleon's army on the Russian front and whose name has been adopted in the description of the complex ligamentous structures of the forefoot. He became famous initially for his description of a novel and extremely rapid technique of forefoot amputation, involving disarticulation across the tarsometatarsal joints without the need for osteotomy. Such amputations became necessary (depending on one's source) as a result either of injuries sustained by riders falling from their horses with a foot caught in stirrups or due to frostbite and gangrene as a consequence of the harsh Russian winter. Despite his skill and reputation, however, he was apparently not a popular man due to his pompous and pugnacious demeanour.

- Although terminology has been confused, the term *Lisfranc joint complex* is now used in clinical practice to describe the intricate complex of ligaments and articulations at the level of the tarsometatarsal joints (illustrated as **G31**). The term *Lisfranc joint* collectively refers to those at the base of the first and second metatarsals (**H32**), and the *Lisfranc ligament* is that which bridges the base of the second metatarsal and medial cuneiform (**H33**). This ligament, as well as the "keystone" wedging of the second metatarsal within the cuneiforms, is of key importance since it provides the only ligamentous support between the first and second metatarsals. Its disruption, which may follow both high velocity and apparently innocent trauma, results in marked weakness of the forefoot articulations and may lead to severe functional instability and subluxation across the tarsometatarsal joints. Unfortunately, plain radiographic findings, especially when acquired non-weightbearing, may be very subtle and such a pattern of injury is frequently missed on initial imaging. The subsequent chronic pain and development of disabling premature degenerative joint disease are therefore a major source of litigation.

Foot *MRI anatomy of the foot—coronal*

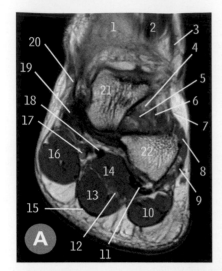

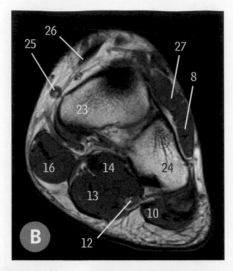

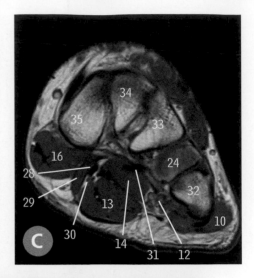

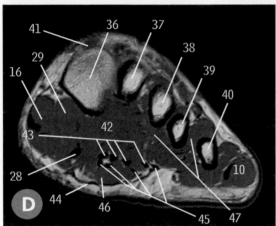

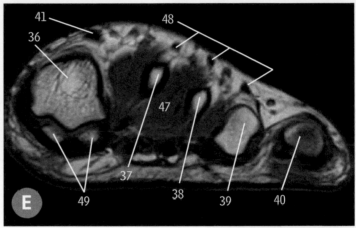

A-F Coronal T1-weighted MR images of the left foot

Dorsal
Medial ◄─────► Lateral
(left)
Plantar

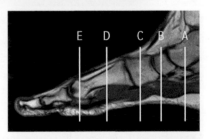

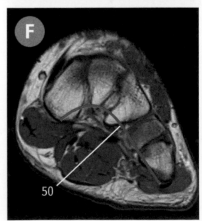

1 Tibia	**27** Extensor hallucis brevis
2 Extensor hallucis longus	**28** Flexor hallucis longus tendon
3 Extensor digitorum longus	**29** Flexor hallucis brevis
4 Sinus tarsi	**30** Deep branches of medial plantar artery and
5 Talocalcaneal interosseous ligament	nerve
6 Cervical ligament	**31** Fibularis (peroneus) longus tendon
7 Extensor retinaculum	**32** Base of fifth metatarsal
8 Extensor digitorum brevis	**33** Lateral
9 Fibularis (peroneus) brevis	**34** Intermediate } cuneiform
10 Abductor digiti minimi	**35** Medial
11 Long plantar ligament (calcaneometatarsal)	**36** First
12 Lateral plantar artery and nerve	**37** Second
13 Flexor digitorum brevis	**38** Third } metatarsal
14 Quadratus plantae	**39** Fourth
15 Plantar aponeurosis (medial part)	**40** Fifth
16 Abductor hallucis	**41** Extensor hallucis longus tendon
17 Medial plantar artery and nerve	**42** Adductor hallucis
18 Tendon of flexor hallucis longus	**43** Flexor digitorum longus tendons
19 Tendon of tibias posterior	**44** Plantar aponeurosis
20 Deltoid ligament (tibiocalcaneal part)	**45** Flexor digitorum brevis tendons
21 Talus	**46** Lumbricals
22 Calcaneus	**47** Interossei
23 Navicular	**48** Extensor digitorum longus tendons
24 Cuboid	**49** Sesamoid bones
25 Great saphenous vein	**50** Transverse arch
26 Tendon of tibialis anterior	

Foot *MRI anatomy of the foot—axial and sagittal*

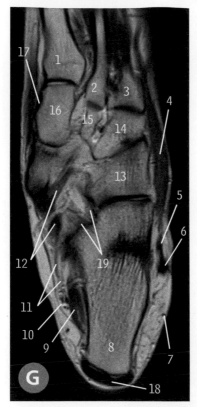

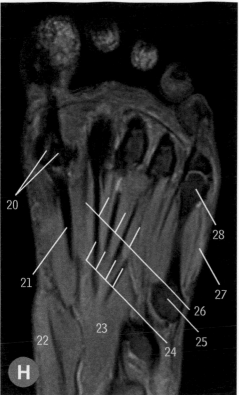

1 First ⎫
2 Second ⎬ metatarsal
3 Third ⎭
4 Extensor digitorum brevis
5 Fibularis (peroneus) brevis tendon
6 Fibularis (peroneus) longus tendon
7 Sural nerve
8 Calcaneus
9 Quadratus plantae
10 Posterior tibial artery and nerve
11 Medial and lateral plantar artery and nerve
12 Flexor digitorum longus tendon
13 Cuboid
14 Lateral ⎫
15 Intermediate ⎬ cuneiform
16 Medial ⎭
17 Tibialis posterior tendon
18 Tendo calcaneus (Achilles tendon)
19 Bifurcate ligament (calcaneonavicular and calcaneocuboid parts)
20 Sesamoid bones
21 Flexor hallucis longus tendon
22 Abductor hallucis
23 Flexor digitorum brevis
24 Flexor digitorum longus tendons
25 Base of fifth metatarsal
26 Lumbricals
27 Abductor digiti minimi
28 Head of fifth metatarsal
29 Talus
30 Tibialis anterior tendon
31 Navicular
32 Medial cuneiform
33 First metatarsal
34 Extensor hallucis longus tendon
35 Proximal ⎫
36 Distal ⎬ phalanx of great toe
37 Flexor hallucis longus tendon
38 Flexor hallucis brevis tendon
39 Flexor hallucis brevis
40 Medial ⎫
41 Lateral ⎬ longitudinal arch

Ⓖ Ⓗ Axial T1-weighted MR images of the left foot, axial view

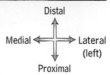

Distal ↑
Medial ←→ Lateral (left)
Proximal ↓

Ⓘ

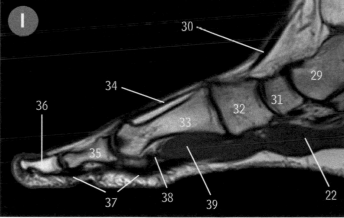

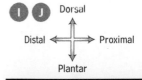

Ⓘ Ⓙ Dorsal ↑
Distal ←→ Proximal
Plantar ↓

Ⓘ Sagittal T1-weighted MR images of the left foot, through the level of the first metatarsal

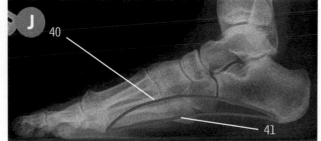

Ⓙ Lateral radiograph of the foot

- Figures **F50** and **J40** and **J41** illustrate the *transverse* and *longitudinal arches* of the foot, which are formed by the configuration of the bones with support from the associated muscles, ligaments and tendons. The arches play a key role in supporting body weight, as well as aiding locomotion via their shock absorptive capacities and ability to provide leverage in a spring-like fashion.

- The transverse arch (**F50**) in reality forms a half-dome in the coronal plane, with a full arch seen when both feet are placed together. The medial longitudinal arch (**J40**) is the higher of the two longitudinal arches and is formed by the calcaneus, talus, navicular, cuneiforms and first three metatarsals. The lateral longitudinal arch is flatter—as evidenced by the mark left by wet feet on a floor—and is formed by the calcaneus, cuboid, fourth and fifth metatarsals.

- Loss of the medial longitudinal arch—which may be acquired or congenital in nature—results in *pes planus* ('flat feet'). In adults, loss of function of the posterior tibialis tendon or muscle, which may occur due to a variety of causes, is an important cause. If untreated, pain, swelling and the development of premature degenerative joint disease may occur.

Foot *Vascular anatomy of the foot and ankle*

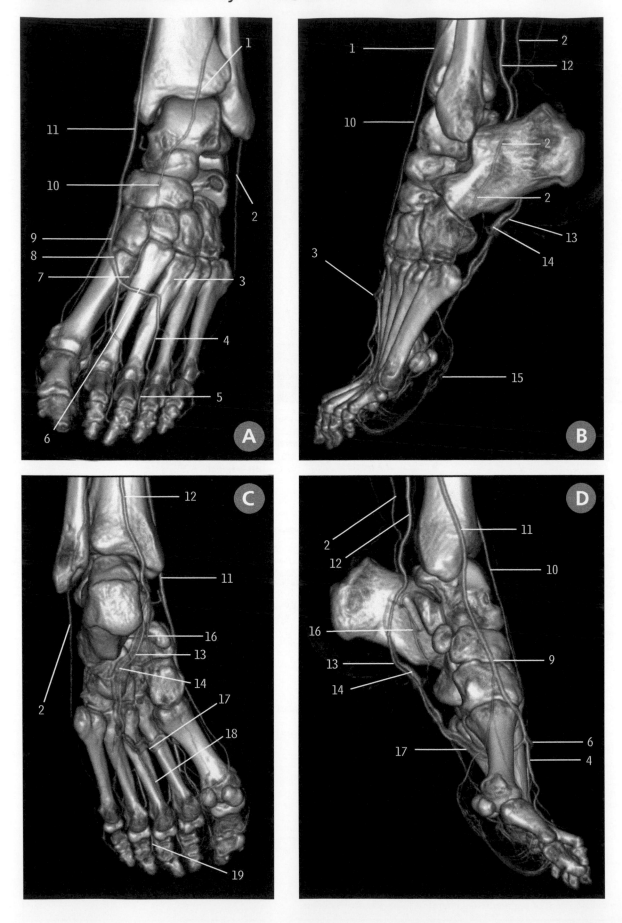

(A)-(D) Volume-rendered CT angiogram images of the left foot and ankle

(A) From above (dorsal surface)

(B) From the lateral side

(C) From posteriorly and below (plantar surface)

(D) From the medial side

1 Anterior tibial artery
2 Fibular (peroneal) artery
3 Lateral marginal vein
4 Metatarsal vein
5 Dorsal digital vein
6 Dorsal venous arch
7 First dorsal metatarsal artery
8 Valve within medial marginal vein
9 Medial marginal vein
10 Dorsalis pedis artery
11 Great saphenous vein
12 Posterior tibial artery
13 Lateral plantar artery
14 Lateral plantar vein
15 Venous plexus of sole
16 Medial plantar artery
17 Plantar arch
18 Metatarsal artery
19 Plantar digital vein

- Figures **A–D** represent CT angiographic images acquired following the injection of intravenous iodinated contrast medium. Because of the timing of image acquisition following injection, early filling of foot veins is also demonstrated (e.g. marginal, plantar and long saphenous veins, **8, 9, 11** and **14**). Certain smaller veins, such as the lateral plantar vein (**D14**), are subsequently seen to fade out above the ankle because of the timing of imaging resulting in a reduced density of contrast medium within the flowing blood. If required, additional imaging following a short delay may be performed to further evaluate the venous system; this is rarely performed, however, due to the lesser importance of venous disease of the foot when compared with that involving the arteries.

- As with the lower leg, considerable variation in arterial and venous anatomy may be observed; in some cases, the posterior tibial artery is is hypoplastic or absent completely, with blood supply to the feet being from branches of the anterior tibial, dorsalis pedis and fibular (peroneal) arteries. This is of clinical importance in the management of patients with peripheral vascular disease (atherosclerosis), who may require surgical intervention.

Foot *Paediatric anatomy*

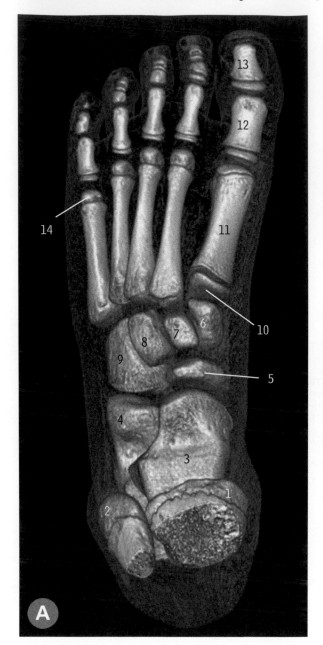

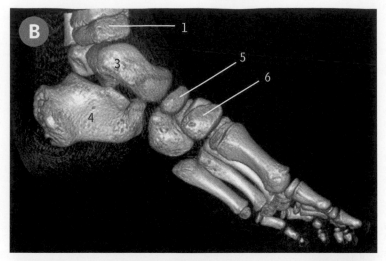

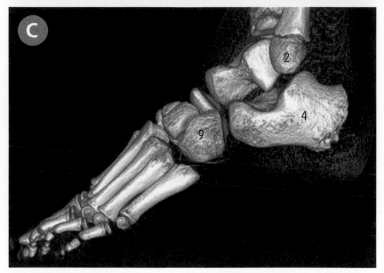

1	Distal tibial epiphysis	**9**	Cuboid
2	Distal fibular epiphysis	**10**	Proximal epiphysis of first
3	Talus		metatarsal
4	Calcaneus	**11**	First metatarsal
5	Navicular	**12**	Proximal } phalanx
6	Medial ⎫	**13**	Distal } phalanx
7	Intermediate ⎬ cuneiform	**14**	Distal metatarsal epiphysis
8	Lateral ⎭		

A–C Volume-rendered CT images of the left foot and ankle

A From above (dorsal surface)   **B** From the medial side   **C** From the lateral side

- Figures **A–C** demonstrate the developing foot in an 8-year-old paediatric patient. Due to the method of computerized reconstruction performed in this case, soft tissues and the foot outline are faintly visible overlying the bones. Numerous centres of ossification within the epiphyses of the longer bones are demonstrated (e.g. **A10**), which subsequently fuse with the adjacent metaphyses. The tarsal bones form from a single centre of ossification: the appearance of increased gaps between them arises from the radiolucency of cartilage from which the bones form rather than from widened joint spaces. In addition, irregularity of certain bones is a normal finding (e.g. calcaneus, **C4**) and should not be confused with pathology.

Appendix

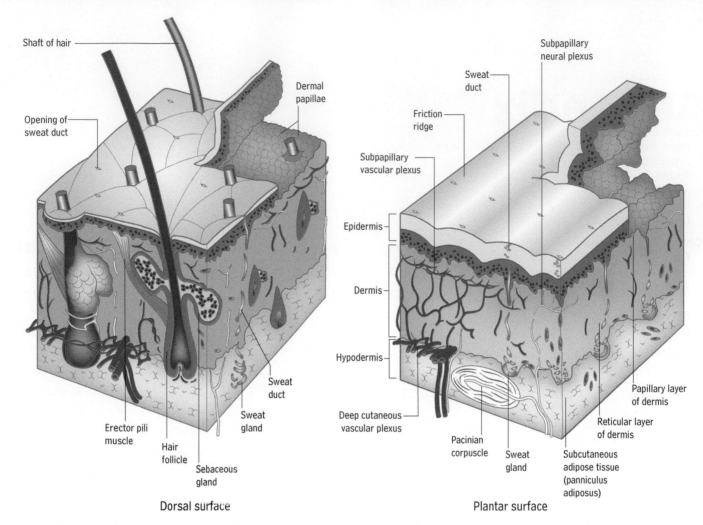

Dorsal surface

Plantar surface

Fig. 1 Schematic diagram comparing the structures present in the thin and hairy dorsal skin and those in the thick, hairless plantar skin of the foot. The epidermis has been partially reflected to show epidermal and dermal papillae.

Skin

The skin of the dorsal and plantar surfaces of the foot differs in appearance and organization (Fig. 1).

Muscles

MUSCLES OF THE GLUTEAL REGION

Gluteus maximus
From the posterior gluteal line of the hip bone, the dorsal surface of the lower part of the sacrum and the side of the coccyx, the sacrotuberous ligament and the fascia over gluteus medius
To the iliotibial tract, with the deep fibres of the lower part attaching to the gluteal tuberosity of the femur
Inferior gluteal nerve, L5, S1, S2
Extension and lateral rotation of the hip joint

Gluteus medius
From the outer surface of the ilium between the posterior and anterior oblique lines
To the lateral surface of the greater trochanter of the femur
Superior gluteal nerve, L4, L5, S1
Abduction and medial rotation of the hip joint and prevention of adduction

Gluteus minimus
From the outer surface of the ilium between the anterior and inferior gluteal lines
To the anterior part of the lateral surface of the greater trochanter of the femur
Superior gluteal nerve, L4, 5, S1
Abduction and medial rotation of the hip joint, and prevention of adduction

Piriformis
From the middle three pieces of the sacrum
To the upper border of the greater trochanter of the femur
Branches from L5, S1, S2
Abduction, lateral rotation and stabilization of the hip joint

Quadratus femoris
From the upper part of the outer border of the ischial tuberosity
To the quadrate tubercle of the intertrochanteric crest of the femur
Nerve to quadratus femoris, L4, L5, S1
Lateral rotation and stabilization of the hip joint

Obturator internus
From the inner surface of the obturator membrane and the adjacent anterolateral pelvic wall
To the greater trochanter of the femur, above and in front of the trochanteric fossa
Nerve to obturator internus, L5, S1, S2
Lateral rotation and stabilization of the hip joint

Gemellus superior and inferior
Superior from the dorsal surface of the ischial spine, inferior from the upper part of the ischial tuberosity
To the superior and inferior borders respectively of obturator internus
Nerves to obturator internus (superior) and quadratus femoris (inferior)
Assists obturator internus

Obturator externus
From the outer surface of the obturator membrane and the ischiopubic ramus
To the trochanteric fossa of the femur
Obturator nerve, L3, L4
Lateral rotator of the thigh

MUSCLES OF THE FRONT OF THE THIGH

Iliacus
From the upper two-thirds of the iliac fossa in the lower abdomen
To the psoas tendon and the femur below and in front of the lesser trochanter
Femoral nerve, L2, L3
Flexor of the hip, assisting psoas major

Psoas major
From the sides of the lumbar vertebrae and intervertebral discs
To the lesser trochanter of the femur
Branches from L1, L2, L3
Flexor of the hip

Tensor fasciae latae
From the anterior 5 cm of the outer lip of the iliac crest
To the iliotibial tract
Superior gluteal nerve, L4, L5, S1
Extensor of the knee and lateral rotator of the leg

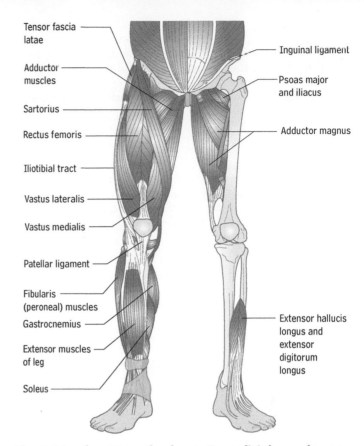

Tensor fascia latae
Adductor muscles
Sartorius
Rectus femoris
Iliotibial tract
Vastus lateralis
Vastus medialis
Patellar ligament
Fibularis (peroneal) muscles
Gastrocnemius
Extensor muscles of leg
Soleus
Inguinal ligament
Psoas major and iliacus
Adductor magnus
Extensor hallucis longus and extensor digitorum longus

Fig. 2 Muscles: From the front. Superficial muscles on the right side of the body; deep muscles on the left side.

Sartorius
From the anterior superior iliac spine
To the upper part of the medial surface of the shaft of the tibia in front of gracilis and semitendinosus
Femoral nerve, L2, L3
Flexor, adductor and lateral rotator of the hip

Rectus femoris
From the anterior inferior iliac spine (straight head) and the ilium above the rim of the acetabulum (reflected head)
To the base of the patella
Femoral nerve, L3, L4
Flexor of the hip and extensor of the knee

Vastus lateralis
From the upper part of the intertrochanteric line of the femur, anterior and inferior borders of the greater trochanter, lateral lip of the gluteal tuberosity and the upper part of the linea aspera
To the lateral border of the patella and the quadriceps tendon
Femoral nerve, L2, L3, L4
Extensor of the knee

Vastus medialis

From the lower part of the intertrochanteric line of the femur, the spiral line, the linea aspera, the upper part of the medial supracondylar line and the tendon of adductor magnus
To the medial border of the patella and the quadriceps tendon
Femoral nerve, L2, L3, L4
Extensor of the knee

Vastus intermedius

From the anterior and lateral surfaces of the upper two-thirds of the shaft of the femur
To the deep part of the quadriceps tendon
Femoral nerve, L2, L3, L4
Extensor of the knee

Articularis genus

From the anterior surface of the femur below vastus intermedius
To the apex of the suprapatellar bursa
Femoral nerve, L3, L4
Retraction of the bursa as the knee extends

MUSCLES OF THE MEDIAL SIDE OF THE THIGH

Pectineus

From the pectineal line of the pubis and bone in front of the line
To the femur on a line from the lesser trochanter to the linea aspera
Femoral nerve, L2, L3
Flexor, adductor and lateral rotator of the hip

Gracilis

From the body of the pubis and ischiopubic ramus
To the upper part of the medial surface of the shaft of the tibia, between sartorius and semitendinosus
Obturator nerve, L2, L3
Flexor, adductor and medial rotator of the thigh

Adductor brevis

From the body and inferior ramus of the pubis
To the shaft of the femur on a line from the lesser trochanter to the linea aspera and to the upper part of the linea
Obturator nerve, L2, L3, L4
Adductor of the thigh

Adductor longus

From the front of the pubis
To the middle part of the linea aspera
Obturator nerve, L2, L3, L4
Adductor of the thigh

Adductor magnus

From the lower lateral part of the ischial tuberosity and the ischiopubic ramus
To the shaft of the femur from the gluteal tuberosity along the linea aspera to the medial supracondylar line and to the adductor tubercle
Obturator nerve, L2, L3, L4 and sciatic nerve, L4, L5, S1
Adductor and lateral rotator of the thigh

MUSCLES OF THE BACK OF THE THIGH

Biceps femoris

From the medial facet of the ischial tuberosity with semimembranosus (long head) and from the linea aspera and lateral supracondylar line of the femur (short head)
To the head of the fibula
Sciatic nerve (tibial part to long head, common fibular (*peroneal*) part to short head), L5, S1
Flexion and lateral rotation of the knee and extension of the hip

Semitendinosus

From the medial facet of the ischial tuberosity, with the long head of biceps
To the upper part of the subcutaneous surface of the tibia, behind gracilis
Sciatic nerve (tibial part), L5, S1
Flexion and medial rotation of the knee and extension of the hip

Semimembranosus

From the lateral facet of the ischial tuberosity
To the groove on the back of the medial condyle of the tibia, with expansions forming the oblique popliteal ligament and the fascia over popliteus
Sciatic nerve (tibial part), L5, S1
Flexion and medial rotation of the knee and extension of the hip

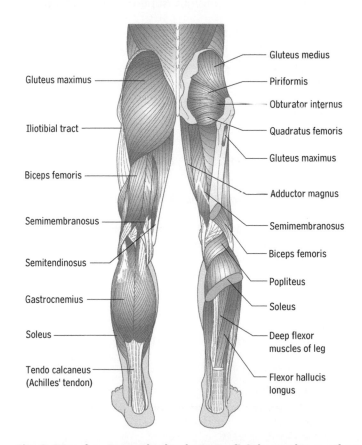

Fig. 3 Muscles: From the back. Superficial muscles on the left side of the body; deep muscles on the right side.

MUSCLES OF THE FRONT OF THE LEG

Tibialis anterior
From the upper two-thirds of the lateral surface of
the tibia and adjoining part of the interosseous
membrane
To the medial surfaces of the medial cuneiform and base
of the first metatarsal
Deep fibular (peroneal) nerve, L4, L5
Dorsiflexion and inversion of the foot

Extensor hallucis longus
From the middle third of the medial surface of the
fibula
To the base of the distal phalanx of the great toe
Deep fibular (peroneal) nerve, L4, L5
Extension of the great toe and dorsiflexion of
the foot

Extensor digitorum longus
From the upper two-thirds of the medial surface of the
fibula
To the four lateral toes by the dorsal digital expansions,
attached to the middle and distal phalanges
Deep fibular (peroneal) nerve, L5, S1
Extension of the second to fifth toes and dorsiflexion of
the foot

Fibularis *(peroneus)* tertius
From the lower third of the medial surface of the fibula,
continuous with extensor digitorum longus
To the shaft of the fifth metatarsal
Deep fibular (peroneal) nerve, L5, S1
Dorsiflexion and eversion of the foot

MUSCLE OF THE DORSUM OF THE FOOT

Extensor digitorum brevis
From the upper surface of the calcaneus
To the base of the proximal phalanx of the great toe
(as extensor hallucis brevis) and the dorsal digital
expansions of the second to fourth toes
Deep fibular (peroneal) nerve, L5, S1
Extension of the first to fourth toes

MUSCLES OF THE LATERAL SIDE OF THE LEG

Fibularis *(peroneus)* longus
From the upper two-thirds of the lateral surface of the
fibula
To the lateral sides of the medial cuneiform and base of
the first metatarsal
Superficial fibular (peroneal) nerve, L5, S1, S2
Plantar flexion and eversion of the foot

Fibularis *(peroneus)* brevis
From the lower two-thirds of the lateral surface of the
fibula
To the tuberosity of the base of the fifth metatarsal
Superficial fibular (peroneal) nerve, L5, S1, S2
Plantar flexion and eversion of the foot

MUSCLES OF THE BACK OF THE LEG

Gastrocnemius
Medial head from the upper posterior part of the
medial condyle of the femur; lateral head from the
lateral surface of the lateral condyle of the femur
To the middle of the posterior surface of the calcaneus
by the tendo calcaneus (in association with soleus)
Tibial nerve, S1, S2
Plantar flexion of the foot and flexion of the knee

Soleus
From the soleal line and upper part of the medial
border of the tibia, a tendinous arch over the
popliteal vessels and tibial nerve and the upper part
of the posterior surface of the fibula
To the tendo calcaneus with gastrocnemius (see above)
Tibial nerve, S1, S2
Plantar flexion of the foot

Plantaris
From the lateral supracondylar line of the femur
To the calcaneus on the medial side of the tendo
calcaneus
Tibial nerve, S1, S2
Plantar flexion of the foot and weak flexion of the knee

Popliteus
From the back of the tibia above the soleal line
To the outer surface of the lateral epicondyle of the
femur
Tibial nerve, L4, L5, S1
Lateral rotation of the femur on the fixed tibia (or
medial rotation of the tibia on the fixed femur); pulls
lateral meniscus backward during flexion of the knee

Tibialis posterior
From the posterior surface of the interosseous membrane
and adjacent posterior surfaces of the tibia and fibula
To the tuberosity of the navicular, with slips to other
tarsal bones (except the talus) and the middle three
metatarsals
Tibial nerve, L4, L5
Plantar flexion and inversion of the foot

Flexor hallucis longus
From the lower two-thirds of the posterior surface of
the fibula
To the plantar surface of the base of the distal phalanx
of the great toe
Tibial nerve, S2, S3
Plantar flexion of the great toe and foot

Flexor digitorum longus
From the medial part of the posterior surface of the
tibia below the soleal line
To the four lateral toes by a tendon to each, reaching
the plantar surface of the base of the distal phalanx
Tibial nerve, S2, S3
Plantar flexion of the four lateral toes and foot

MUSCLES OF THE SOLE OF THE FOOT

FIRST LAYER (Fig. 4)

Abductor hallucis
From the medial process of the calcanean tuberosity and the plantar aponeurosis
To the medial side of the proximal phalanx of the great toe
Medial plantar nerve, S2, S3
Abduction and plantar flexion of the great toe

Flexor digitorum brevis
From the medial process of the calcanean tuberosity and the deep surface of the central part of the plantar aponeurosis
To the lateral four toes by a tendon to each; the tendon divides into two slips (to allow the flexor digitorum longus tendon to pass between them), which are attached to the sides of the middle phalanx
Medial plantar nerve, S2, S3
Plantar flexion of the four lateral toes

Abductor digiti minimi
From the lateral and medial processes of the calcanean tuberosity and the plantar aponeurosis
To the lateral side of the base of the proximal phalanx of the fifth toe (with flexor digiti minimi brevis)
Lateral plantar nerve, S2, S3
Abduction and plantar flexion of the fifth toe

SECOND LAYER (Fig. 5)

Quadratus plantae (flexor accessorius)
*From the (concave) medial surface of the calcaneus and from the plantar surface of the calcaneus in front of the lateral process of the tuberosity
To the lateral border of flexor digitorum longus before the division into four tendons
Lateral plantar nerve, S2, S3
Assistance with plantar flexion of the four lateral toes

Lumbricals
First lumbrical from the medial border of the first tendon of flexor digitorum longus
Second, third and fourth lumbricals from the four adjoining tendons of flexor digitorum longus
To the medial sides of the dorsal digital expansions of the tendons of extensor digitorum longus
First lumbrical—medial plantar nerve; second, third and fourth lumbricals by the lateral plantar nerve, S2, S3
Plantar flexion at the four lateral metatarsophalangeal joints and extension at interphalangeal joints
Tendons of flexor digitorum longus and flexor hallucis longus

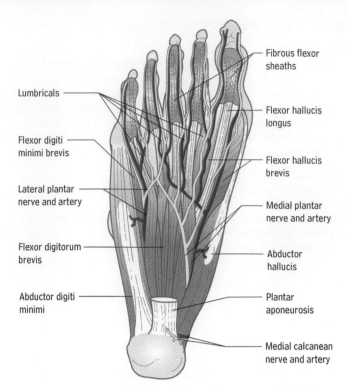

Fig. 4 Muscles of the sole of the right foot: first layer. For dissection see p. 92.

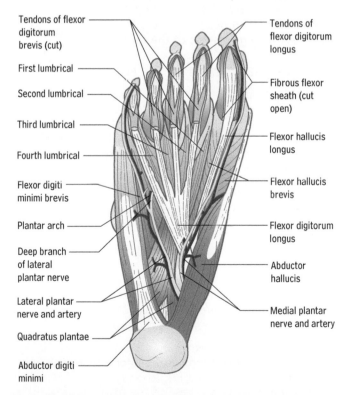

Fig. 5 Muscles of the sole of the right foot: second layer. For dissection see p. 93.

THIRD LAYER (Fig. 6)

Flexor hallucis brevis
From the plantar surface of the cuboid and lateral cuneiform
By a tendon to each side of the base of the proximal phalanx of the great toe, the medial tendon joining with that of abductor hallucis and the lateral with adductor hallucis; there is a sesamoid bone in each tendon
Medial plantar nerve, S2, S3
Plantar flexion of the metatarsophalangeal joint of the great toe

Adductor hallucis
Oblique head from the bases of the second, third and fourth metatarsals
Transverse head from the plantar metatarsophalangeal ligaments of the third, fourth and fifth toes
To the lateral side of the base of the proximal phalanx of the great toe, with part of flexor hallucis brevis
Lateral plantar nerve, S2, S3
Adduction of the great toe

Flexor digiti minimi brevis
From the plantar surface of the base of the fifth metatarsal
To the lateral side of the base of proximal phalanx of the fifth toe, with abductor digiti minimi
Lateral plantar nerve, S2, S3
Plantar flexion of the metatarsophalangeal joint of the fifth toe

FOURTH LAYER (Fig. 7)

Dorsal interosseous (four)
From adjacent sides of the bodies of the metatarsals
To the bases of proximal phalanges and the dorsal digital expansions; first and second to the medial and lateral sides of the second toe; third and fourth to the lateral sides of the third and fourth toes
Lateral plantar nerve, S2, S3
Plantar flexion of the metatarsophalangeal joints and extension (dorsiflexion) of the interphalangeal joints of the second, third and fourth toes; abduction of the same toes

Plantar interosseous (three)
From the bases and medial sides of the third, fourth and fifth metatarsals
To the medial sides of the bases of the proximal phalanges and dorsal digital expansions of the corresponding toes
Lateral plantar nerve, S2, S3
Plantar flexion of the metatarsophalangeal joints and extension (dorsiflexion) of the interphalangeal joints of the third, fourth and fifth toes; adduction of the same toes
Tendons of tibialis posterior and fibularis (*peroneus*) longus

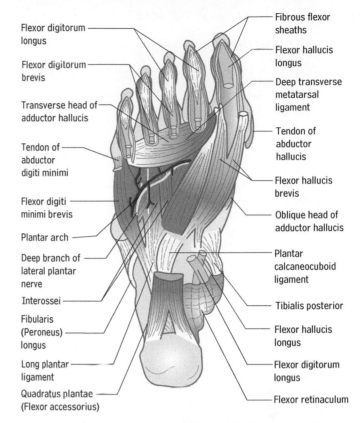

Fig. 6 Muscles of the sole of the right foot: third layer. For dissection see p. 94.

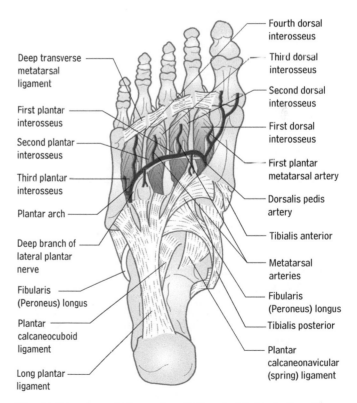

Fig. 7 Muscles of the sole of the right foot: fourth layer. For dissection see p. 95.

Nerves

BRANCHES OF THE LUMBAR PLEXUS (Fig. 8)

Muscular T12, L1, L2, L3, L4 to psoas major and minor, quadratus lumborum and iliacus

Iliohypogastric and ilioinguinal L1 to parts of internal oblique and transversus abdominis in anterior abdominal wall

Genitofemoral L1, L2, giving off
  Genital branch (to cremaster muscle of spermatic cord)
  Femoral branch

Lateral cutaneous of thigh L2, L3

Femoral L2, L3, L4, giving off
  Nerve to pectineus
  Anterior division, giving off
    Intermediate femoral cutaneous
    Medial femoral cutaneous
    Nerve to sartorius
  Posterior division, giving off
    Saphenous
    Nerves to quadriceps femoris

Obturator L2, L3, L4, giving off
  Anterior branch
    Muscular to adductor longus, adductor brevis and gracilis
  Posterior branch
    Muscular to obturator externus and adductor magnus

Accessory obturator (occasional) L3, L4 to pectineus

BRANCHES OF THE SACRAL PLEXUS

Superior gluteal L4, L5, S1, to gluteus medius, gluteus minimus and tensor fasciae latae

Inferior gluteal L5, S1, S2, to gluteus maximus

Nerve to piriformis S1, S2

Nerve to quadratus femoris and gemellus inferior L4, L5, S1

Nerve to obturator internus and gemellus superior L5, S1, S2

Posterior femoral cutaneous S2, S3

Sciatic nerve L4, L5, S1, S2, S3 giving off
  Muscular branches to biceps, semimembranosus, semitendinosus and part of adductor magnus
  Tibial nerve—see below
  Common fibular (*peroneal*) nerve—see below

Perforating cutaneous, pudendal and other pelvic and perineal branches

BRANCHES OF THE TIBIAL NERVE L4, L5, S1, S2, S3 (Fig. 9)

Muscular to gastrocnemius, plantaris, soleus, popliteus, tibialis posterior, flexor digitorum longus and flexor hallucis longus

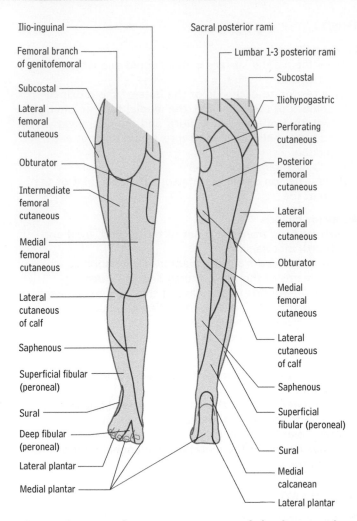

Fig. 8 Diagram of cutaneous nerves of the front and back of the right lower limb.

Sural (ending as lateral dorsal cutaneous and then dorsal digital to lateral side of fifth toe)
Medial calcanean
Medial plantar—see below
Lateral plantar—see below

BRANCHES OF THE COMMON FIBULAR (*PERONEAL*) NERVE L4, L5, S1, S2

Recurrent
Lateral cutaneous of calf
Fibular (peroneal) communicating

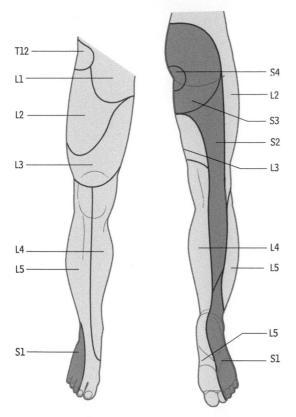

Fig. 9 Diagram of dermatomes of the front and back of the right lower limb. (A dermatome is the area of skin supplied by any one spinal nerve.) Note that both the dorsum and sole of the foot are supplied by L5 and S1 dermatomes.

Superficial fibular (peroneal), giving off
  Muscular to fibularis (*peroneus*) longus and fibularis
    (peroneus) brevis
  Medial branch (medial dorsal cutaneous), giving off
    Dorsal digital
  Lateral branch (intermediate dorsal cutaneous),
    giving off
    Dorsal digital
Deep fibular (peroneal), giving off
  Muscular to tibialis anterior, extensor hallucis longus,
    extensor digitorum longus and fibularis (*peroneus*)
    tertius
  Lateral terminal, to extensor digitorum brevis
  Medial terminal, giving off
    Dorsal digital (to first cleft)

BRANCHES OF THE MEDIAL PLANTAR NERVE L4, L5, S1

Trunk giving off
  Nerve to abductor hallucis
  Nerve to flexor digitorum brevis
Proper plantar digital nerve of great toe, giving off
  Nerve to flexor hallucis brevis
First common plantar digital nerve, giving off
  Nerve to first lumbrical
  Proper plantar digital nerves of first cleft
Second common plantar digital nerve, giving off
  Proper plantar digital nerves of second cleft
Third common plantar digital nerve, giving off
  Proper plantar digital nerves of third cleft

BRANCHES OF THE LATERAL PLANTAR NERVE S1, S2

Trunk, giving off
  Nerve to quadratus plantae
  Nerve to abductor digiti minimi
Superficial branch, giving off
  Fourth common plantar digital nerve, giving off
    Proper plantar digital nerves of fourth cleft
  Proper plantar digital nerve of fifth toe, giving off
    Nerve to flexor digiti minimi brevis
    Nerve to third plantar interosseous
    Nerve to fourth dorsal interosseous
Deep branch, giving off
  Nerve to adductor hallucis
  Nerves to second, third and fourth lumbricals
  Nerves to first, second and third dorsal interossei
  Nerves to first and second plantar interossei

Regional anaesthesia
for foot and ankle

- Popliteal Block
- Ankle Block
- Midfoot Field Block
- Common Digital Block

Advantages
- Most foot and ankle surgery can be performed in the day care setting.
- A combination of regional or field block with or without general anaesthesia allows faster patient recovery and better postoperative analgesia.

POPLITEAL BLOCK

A popliteal block essentially blocks two terminal branches of the sciatic nerve but has to be combined with a saphenous nerve block to ensure complete effectiveness of block technique. The nerves can be identified using the nerve stimulator (1) or, more easily, using the ultrasound (2) technique as described below.

Indications

For surgery on the ankle or foot, this block can be used as the sole anaesthetic or in conjunction with general or spinal anaesthesia for postoperative analgesia. If a tourniquet is required, a calf tourniquet should be used.

Contraindications

1. Patient refusal

2. Infection of the site of block

3. Coagulopathy

Precautions

As surgery on the forefoot can be easily performed under an ankle block; a popliteal block in these cases is not necessary. It will cause foot drop, which may delay patient mobilization or discharge.

Anatomy

The predominant nerve innervating the lower limb below the knee is the sciatic nerve and its branches. The saphenous nerve is the only sensory contribution below the knee.

The sciatic nerve divides at a variable distance proximal to the popliteal crease into the tibial and common fibular (peroneal) nerve branches.

The saphenous nerve is a branch of the femoral nerve from its posterior division. It leaves the femoral triangle at its lower angle and passes across the front of the femoral artery in the subsartorial canal to reach the medial side of the vessel. It leaves the canal by passing beneath the posterior border of sartorius and becomes superficial posterior and lateral to the knee joint, then travels the leg distally along with the great saphenous vein as far as the medial side of the foot).

(1) NERVE STIMULATOR-GUIDED TECHNIQUE

Although various approaches to the nerves situated in the popliteal fossa have been described, the preferable one is the posterior approach. This approach is less painful to the patient as the needle passes only through skin and adipose tissue on its way to the nerves.

Equipment and drugs

1. Nerve stimulator (e.g. B Braun Stimuplex)

2. Insulated 50 mm needle

3. Local anaesthetic: Use 0.5% levobupivacaine for anaesthesia and 0.25% if the block is done only for postoperative analgesia.

Procedure (Fig. 10)

After intravenous access is established and appropriate monitoring applied, the patient lies in a prone position with a pillow placed underneath the leg so that the knee becomes slightly flexed.

A line is drawn on the skin along the popliteal crease and along this line the tendon of biceps is felt on the lateral side of the fossa and marked. Similarly, the tendon of semitendinosus is felt and marked on the medial side.

The line marking the popliteal crease between these tendons is divided and a perpendicular line drawn cephalad from this point.

A point on the perpendicular line is marked 7 cm from the popliteal crease line and the needle insertion point is 1 cm lateral to this point.

An intradermal wheal of local anaesthetic is injected at this point.

A 5 cm stimulating needle is then inserted perpendicular to the skin and initial stimulating current set at 1 mA, frequency 2 Hz.

Nerve stimulation should be elicited within 1.5–2.5 cm.

With this approach, the common fibular (peroneal) nerve is often first identified, causing dorsiflexion of the foot.

Once the needle is adjusted so that a twitch may be found at 0.3–0.5 mA, 10 ml of local anaesthetic is injected after excluding intravascular needle placement by careful aspiration, the twitch should disappear immediately.

The needle should then be redirected to stimulate the second nerve, by either moving it medially to locate the tibial nerve (if the common fibular (peroneal) nerve was found first) or laterally to locate the common fibular (peroneal) nerve (if the tibial nerve was found first).

When the other nerve is located, another 10 ml of local anaesthetic is injected.

Complications

1. Nerve damage

2. Intravascular injection leading to local anaesthetic toxicity

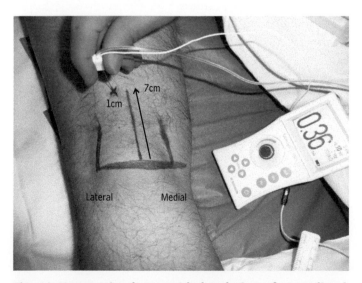

Fig. 10 Nerve stimulator-guided technique for popliteal block.

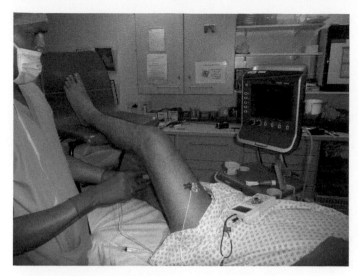

Fig. 11 Ultrasound technique for popliteal block

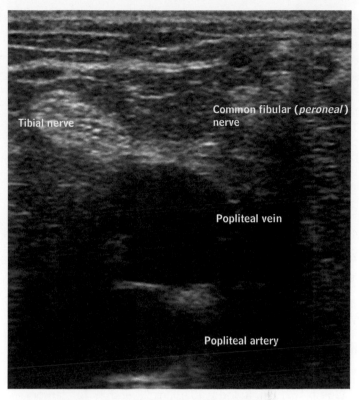

Fig. 12 Ultrasound image of popliteal fossa.

(2) ULTRASOUND TECHNIQUE

A popliteal block can be safely and easily done using ultrasound. Indications, contraindications and complications are similar to the nerve stimulator-guided technique.

Equipment and drugs

1. Ultrasound machine with high frequency linear probe

2. Probe cover and jelly

3. Nerve stimulator (e.g. B Braun Stimuplex)

4. Insulated 100 mm needle

5. Local anaesthetic. Use 0.5% levobupivacaine for anaesthesia and 0.25% if the block is done only for postoperative analgesia.

Procedure (Figs 11 and 12)

After intravenous access is established and appropriate monitoring applied, the patient lies supine with leg elevated and resting on a support.

The ultrasound probe is placed behind the knee just above the popliteal crease so that a transverse (cross-sectional) image of the popliteal artery and vein superior to it may be observed.

Nerves lay superficially to the blood vessels and the tibial nerve (largest) is identified first; then the common fibular (*peroneal*) nerve, which is seen to converge with the tibial nerve when the probe is moved cephalad, is identified.

Once the nerves have been clearly identified, a needle is inserted in the scanning plane so that the entire needle can be observed on the screen live, as it approaches the nerves; then, 20 ml of local anaesthetic is injected to surround the nerves.

Complications of this procedure are similar to nerve stimulator-guided procedure.

ANKLE BLOCK

The ankle block is a simple block to perform that targets the terminal branches of the sciatic and femoral nerves. Complete ankle block requires five injections; mild sedation, therefore, may improve patient comfort during block performance.

Indications

This block can be used as an anaesthetic technique for surgery on the forefoot. It can also be used for postoperative analgesia for surgery on the midfoot done under general anaesthesia, since most of these types of surgery need a thigh tourniquet.

Contraindications

1. Patient refusal

2. Infection at the site of block

3. Coagulopathy

Anatomy

The five nerves to block are:

The saphenous nerve, which arises from the femoral nerve.

The tibial, superficial and deep fibular (*peroneal*), and sural nerves, which are branches of the sciatic nerve.

(See p.152, Fig. 8 and p.163, Figs 22 and 23 for sensory innervation of the ankle).

Four of the five nerves lie very close to blood vessels:

1. The saphenous nerve lies close to the great saphenous vein in the subcutaneous tissue just in front of the medial malleolus.

2. The tibial nerve lies behind the posterior tibial artery, posterior to the medial malleolus, halfway between the malleolus and the tendo calcaneus (*Achilles tendon*).

3. The deep fibular (*peroneal*) nerve runs with the dorsalis pedis artery on the anterior aspect of the ankle.

4. The sural nerve lies on the lateral side of the tendo calcaneus in close proximity to the short saphenous vein.

The superficial fibular (*peroneal*) nerve begins on the lateral aspect of the neck of the fibula and descends to a point on the anterior border of the leg at which it pierces the deep fascia and divides into medial and lateral branches which diverge in the subcutaneous plane between the two malleoli.

Equipment and drugs

1. 23G hypodermic needle

2. 2% chlorhexidine

3. 20 ml of 0.5% levobupivacaine

Procedure

1. The saphenous nerve (Fig. 13)—subcutaneous infiltration above and slightly anterior to the medial malleolus

2. The tibial nerve (Fig. 14)—behind medial malleolus, posterior to the posterior tibial artery under the sustentaculum tali

3. The sural nerve (Fig. 15)—four-finger breadths above the lateral malleolus in the subcutaneous plane toward the tendo calcaneus

4. The superficial fibular (*peroneal*) nerve (Fig. 16)—subcutaneous infiltration between the two malleoli. Start in the midline and inject on either side.

5. The deep fibular (*peroneal*) nerve (Fig. 17)—on the anterior aspect of the ankle, inject either side of the dorsalis pedis artery.

Complications

1. Intravascular injection

2. May effect mobilization if proprioception is affected

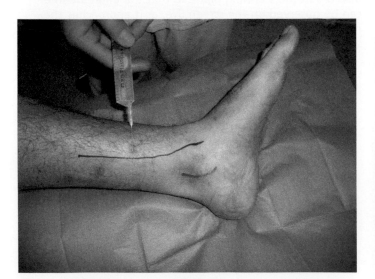

Fig. 13 Saphenous nerve block.

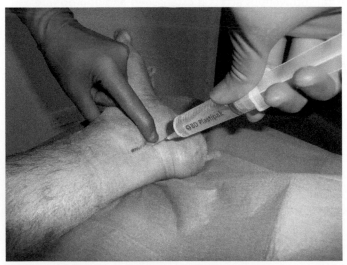

Fig. 14 Tibial nerve block.

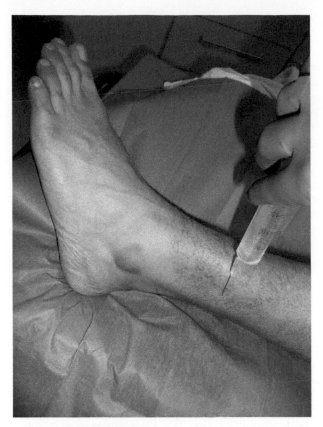

Fig. 15 Sural nerve block.

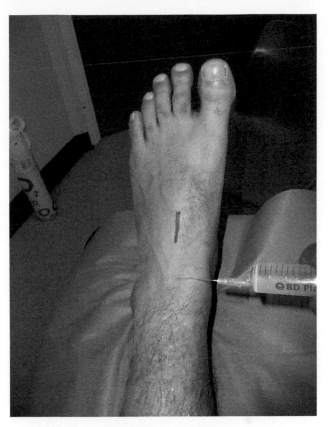

Fig. 16 Superficial fibular (*peroneal*) nerve block.

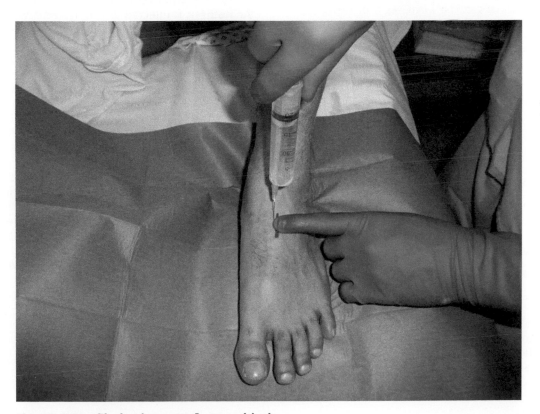

Fig. 17 Deep fibular (*peroneal*) nerve block.

MIDFOOT FIELD BLOCK

The midfoot field block is a simple block to perform. There is no requirement for a nerve stimulator or ultrasound guidance. This technique has proven to be very reliable for surgery on up to three rays of the forefoot. Limbers and associates reported a 100% success rate in 42 patients in a day care environment undergoing forefoot surgery. There were no conversions to a general anaesthetic, and the patients were sedated at the time of block insertion. The surgery was undertaken under an ankle tourniquet. Previous studies have shown similar results with 98% to 100% success rates.

Other midfoot blocks have been described and are known eponymously as the *Sharrock* and *Mayo* blocks. The midtarsal block described by *Sharrock* involves a block of the deep fibular (*peroneal*) nerve and posterior tibial nerve.

The deep fibular (*peroneal*) nerve lies lateral to the dorsalis pedis artery that is located by palpation.

The posterior tibial nerve is anaesthetised by palpating the posterior tibial artery and injecting posterior to it.

These two nerve blocks are supplemented by a subcutaneous field block, anaesthetising the superficial fibular (*peroneal*) and saphenous nerves.

The *Mayo* block involves infiltration of a local anaesthetic ring block in the tissues proximal to the surgical site. A wheal is raised proximal to the first digital interspace after which the needle is advanced in a plantar direction and additional anaesthetic injected. The needle is then withdrawn and directed medially from the dorsal surface to raise a wheal.

These blocks are intermediate procedures between anatomical nerve blocks at the ankle, as previously described, and local infiltration. The block described here, is a modification of the midfoot block as described by *Ptaszek and associates,* it is easy to perform and can be combined with controlled intravenous sedation if required.

Indications

1. Bunion surgery

2. First metatarsophalangeal joint fusion

3. Forefoot surgery (maximum three toes)

Contraindications

1. Patient refusal

2. Infection at the site of block

3. Coagulopathy

4. Allergy to anaesthetic agents

Anatomy

The Great Toe of the foot is supplied by branches of four main nerves, three dorsal and one plantar: dorsally—the superficial fibular (*peroneal*) nerve, saphenous nerve and deep fibular (*peroneal*) nerve; plantar—the medial plantar nerve.

The superficial fibular (*peroneal*) nerve divides at the level of the ankle into medial and lateral branches. The medial branch divides into two dorsal digital nerves: one branch supplies the medial side of the great toe and the other the adjacent sides of the second and third toes. It communicates with the saphenous nerve and deep fibular (*peroneal*) nerve, the terminal branch of which supplies sensation to the dorsum of the first web space (p.163, Fig. 22, A, B).

The medial plantar nerve is a branch of the tibial nerve and supplies the medial–plantar aspect of the great toe (p.163, Fig. 23 A, B). The common plantar digital nerves, which divide to supply the remaining plantar aspect of the medial three and a half toes, are also branches of the medial plantar nerve.

Equipment and drugs

1. 23G hypodermic needle

2. 2% chlorhexidine

3. 5–20 ml of 2% lignocaine without adrenaline (maximum dose of 4.5 mg/kg)

Procedure

Prior to block insertion, the patient may be sedated with monitored intravenous sedation.

The first injection site (Fig. 18) is at the level of the tarsometatarsal joint medially.

The needle is advanced in the subcutaneous plane from dorsal to plantar until the plantar skin is tented. Anaesthetic is injected as the needle is withdrawn.

The saphenous and medial plantar nerves are blocked at this point.

A small amount of anaesthetic is also injected subperiosteally into the first metatarsal.

The second injection site (Fig. 19) is into the first web space to block the medial terminal branch of the deep fibular (*peroneal*) nerve.

Along with infiltration of the web space, subperiosteal infiltration of the lateral first metatarsal is also undertaken.

The third injection site (Fig. 20) is on the plantar surface, just proximal to the metatarsophalangeal joint and blocks the plantar digital nerves.

If surgery to other toes is planned, the lesser rays are blocked with supplementary common digital blocks. Practically however, it is difficult to extend this block beyond three-toe surgery since the volume of anaesthetic required exceeds the toxic dose.

Complications

1. Intravascular injection

2. Failure of the block

3. Neuropraxia

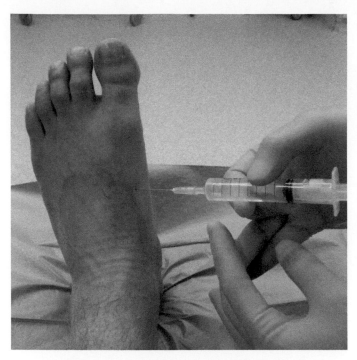

Fig. 18 First injection site for midfoot field block.

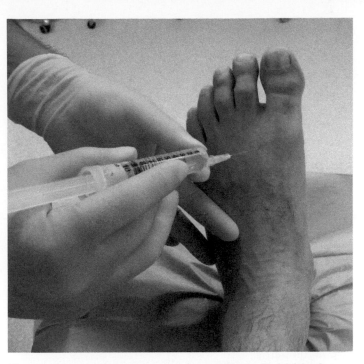

Fig. 19 Second injection site for midfoot field block.

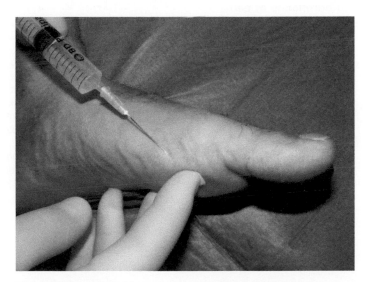

Fig. 20 Third injection site for midfoot field block.

THE COMMON DIGITAL BLOCK

The nerve supply to the lesser toes, 2, 3, 4, 5, is identical to that of the fingers. In the foot, four nerves supply each digit, two dorsal (dorsal digital nerves) and two plantar (proper plantar digital nerves). The dorsal nerves are branches of the superficial fibular (*peroneal*) nerve and the plantar nerves are from divisions of the medial and lateral plantar nerves (p.163, Figs A,B).

The common digital block is preferred to using a ring block because it causes less soft tissue swelling and tension, and it does not compromise surgical dissection. An ankle or toe tourniquet can be used with this block.

Indications

1. Nail surgery

2. Interphalangeal joint fusion

3. Flexor tenotomy

Contraindications

1. Infection at site of block

2. Coagulopathy

3. Patient refusal

4. Allergy to anaesthetic

Equipment and drugs

1. 23G hypodermic needle

2. 2% chlorhexidine

3. 2.5 ml of 1% lignocaine without adrenaline at each injection site (maximum dose of 4.5 ml /kg)

Procedure (Fig. 21)

The needle is inserted in the web space at the level of the metatarsophalangeal joint and advanced vertically until it tents the plantar skin.

The needle is then slowly withdrawn and approximately 2.5 ml of local anaesthetic injected.

This procedure is then repeated on the opposite side of the same toe.

As with digital block in the fingers, co-administration of epinephrine must be avoided since this can cause spasm of the end arteries that supply the digits, resulting in ischaemia and even necrosis.

Complications

1. Intravascular injection

2. Failure to block

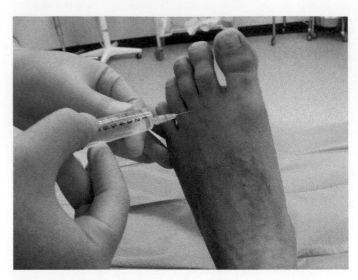

Fig. 21 Common digital block.

Bibliography

Latifzai, K., Sites, B.D., Koval, K.J., 2008. Orthopaedic anaesthesia: Part 2. Common techniques for regional anaesthesia in orthopaedics. *Bull. NYU Hosp. Jt. Dis.* 66, 306–316.

Limbers, J.B., Hutchinson, J.R.M., Obey, P., et al., 2004. Scarf osteotomy as a day case procedure. The patient's perspective. *J. Bone Surg. (Br.) Proceedings* 87-B, 373.

Ptaszek, A.J., Morris, S.G., Brodsky, J.W., 1999. Midfoot field block anaesthesia with monitored intravenous sedation in forefoot surgery. *Foot Ankle Internat.* 20, 583–6.

Sharrock, N., Waller, J., Fierro, L., 1986. Midtarsal block for surgery of the forefoot. *Br. J. Anaesthesia* 58, 37–40.

Worell, J.B., Barbour, G., 1996. The Mayo block: an efficacious block for hallux and First metatarsal surgery. *AANAJ* 64, 146–152.

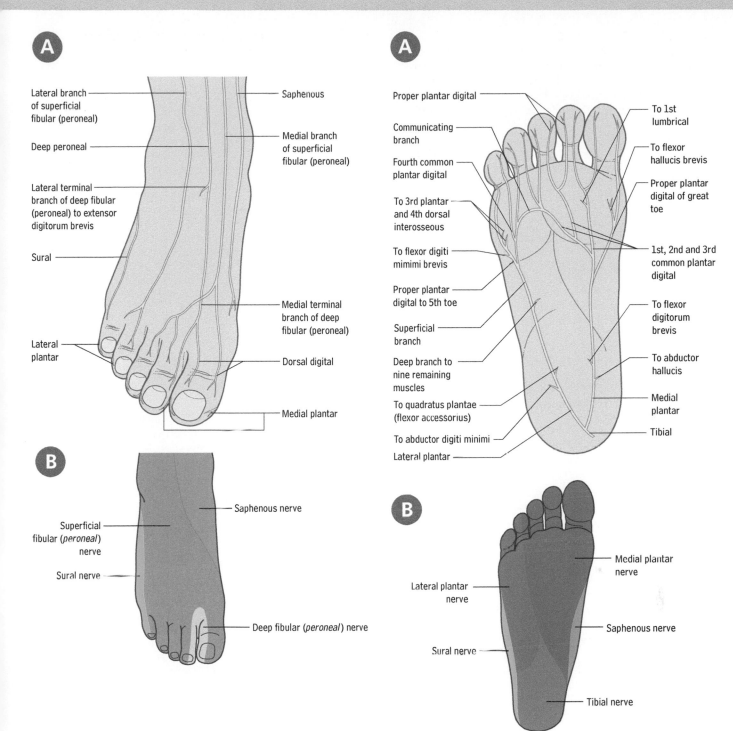

A

Lateral branch of superficial fibular (peroneal)

Deep peroneal

Lateral terminal branch of deep fibular (peroneal) to extensor digitorum brevis

Sural

Lateral plantar

Saphenous

Medial branch of superficial fibular (peroneal)

Medial terminal branch of deep fibular (peroneal)

Dorsal digital

Medial plantar

A

Proper plantar digital

Communicating branch

Fourth common plantar digital

To 3rd plantar and 4th dorsal interosseous

To flexor digiti mimimi brevis

Proper plantar digital to 5th toe

Superficial branch

Deep branch to nine remaining muscles

To quadratus plantae (flexor accessorius)

To abductor digiti minimi

Lateral plantar

To 1st lumbrical

To flexor hallucis brevis

Proper plantar digital of great toe

1st, 2nd and 3rd common plantar digital

To flexor digitorum brevis

To abductor hallucis

Medial plantar

Tibial

B

Superficial fibular (peroneal) nerve

Sural nerve

Saphenous nerve

Deep fibular (peroneal) nerve

B

Lateral plantar nerve

Sural nerve

Medial plantar nerve

Saphenous nerve

Tibial nerve

Fig. 22 A B
Fig. 23 A B   **Sensory innervation of the ankle**

The lymphatic system

GENERAL KEY POINTS

The lymphatic system has four major functions:
1. **Produce, store** and **recirculate lymphocytes**, cells mainly responsible for immune response in the body.
2. **Store macrophages** (phagocytes).
3. **Drain** surplus **tissue fluid** to the bloodstream.
4. **Transport** absorbed **fat** from the intestine to the bloodstream.

The **combined fluid product** is known as **lymph**.

- **Lymph is drained** from areas of tissue **via** very **fine** threadlike lymphatic vessels (**lymphatics**), that are thin walled, **similar to veins,** and **have valves** to ensure **one-way flow**.
- **Lymph flow** is chiefly **maintained by external pressure** on the delicate-walled lymphatic vessels by surrounding tissue structures.
- **Lymphatics connect to main trunks** and are **interrupted** en route **by lymphoid organs** and **nodes,** which act as filters.
- **Afferent lymphatic vessels** carry unfiltered lymph **into a node**.
- **Efferent lymphatic vessels** carry filtered lymph **out of a node**.
- **Several main lymphatic trunks** converge towards their venous junction (cervical lymphovenous portals), returning lymph to the venous bloodstream.

There are normally **three** trunks on the **right side** of the body and **four** on the **left**.

Right-sided trunks	Left-sided trunks
Right jugular trunk	Left jugular trunk
Right subclavian trunk	Left subclavian trunk
Right bronchomediastinal trunk	Left bronchomediastinal trunk
	Thoracic duct

- The **main lymphoid organs of the body** are the **tonsils, spleen, thymus** and **lymph nodes,** of which some 400–450 are present in the normal adult.
- Lymph **nodes** are **sited regionally** and may be found as **singleton, pairs** or in distinct multiple **cluster groups** (Fig. 24).
- **Nodes** are usually **small, ovoid** or **kidney** (reniform) **in shape** and vary between 0.1 and 2.5 cm in length.
- **Some nodes,** but **not all,** may be **palpable** in their **normal state,** but particularly so when diseased.

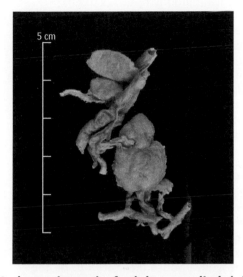

5 cm

Fig. 24 A cluster (group) of adult upper limb left axillary (lateral) lymph nodes with associated vessels. They are shown actual size as presented at dissection and are typical of normal lymph node appearance in the human body.

LOWER LIMB LYMPHATICS—KEY POINTS

- **Not many lymph nodes** are located in the **limbs**.
- The leg and superficial gluteal region, infra-umbilical abdominal wall and perineum have only about **20 recognized lymph nodes**. This does not include the intra-pelvic and intra-abdominal, iliac, lateral caval and aortic groups of nodes, into which the limb lymphatics drain.
- The **lymphatic drainage** of the **lower limb** is via a network of **superficial** and **deep** efferent lymphatic vessels, some of which may directly interconnect, or unite by an afferent vessel to a particular lymph node or group (cluster of nodes).
- Essentially, **superficial** lymphatics of the lower limb accompany superficial **veins**, whereas **deep** lymphatics accompany **arteries**.
- Both **superficial** and **deep** lymphatic networks of the lower limb **drain** in a **distal** (foot) **to proximal** (thigh/groin) limb direction.
- The intra-abdominal **right-side** superior **lateral caval group of lymph nodes** and opposite **left-side** superior **lateral aortic group of lymph** nodes are stated to be **the terminal groups** of nodes **for the lower limbs**.
- From the **lateral caval** and **aortic** groups of nodes, **lymph flows** through the **bilateral lumbar trunks**, their **confluence (cisterna chyli)** and then into the **thoracic duct**.
- **Lymph** finally **returns to** the **venous bloodstream** via a **lymphovenous portal** situated on the **left-side root of neck**, where the thoracic duct drains into the **junction** of the **internal jugular** and **subclavian vein**.
- The **inguinal nodes** are of **key importance** for **lower limb**. They may become enlarged due to infection of the foot (e.g. infected ingrowing toenail) or through involvement by tumour (e.g. leg melanoma).

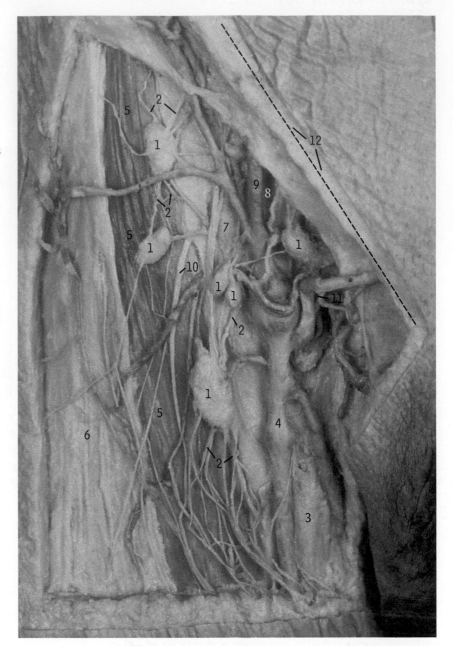
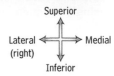

Fig. 25 Superficial dissection of the right upper thigh femoral (triangle) region, displaying lymph nodes and associated lymphatic vessels in situ, from the front

1 Superficial inguinal lymph nodes	7 Femoral artery
2 Lymphatic vessels	8 Femoral vein
3 Fascia overlying adductor longus	9 Superficial epigastric vein
4 Great saphenous vein	10 Saphenous nerve
5 Sartorius	11 Superficial external pudendal artery and vein
6 Iliotibial tract	12 Position of inguinal ligament

Lymph nodes draining the lower limbs

Abdominal lymph nodes
Parietal lymph nodes
  Left lumbar nodes
    Lateral aortic nodes
  Right lumbar nodes
    Lateral caval nodes

Pelvic lymph nodes
Parietal lymph nodes
    Common iliac nodes
    External iliac nodes
    Internal iliac nodes
    Gluteal nodes
      Superior nodes
      Inferior nodes

Lower limb lymph nodes
Inguinal lymph nodes
    Superficial inguinal nodes
      Superomedial nodes
      Superolateral nodes
      Inferior nodes
    Deep inguinal nodes
      (Proximal node)
      (Intermediate node)
      Distal node
    Popliteal nodes
      Superficial nodes
      Deep nodes
    (Anterior tibial node)
    (Posterior tibial node)
    (Fibular [peroneal] node)

note: (( )) structures inconsistent

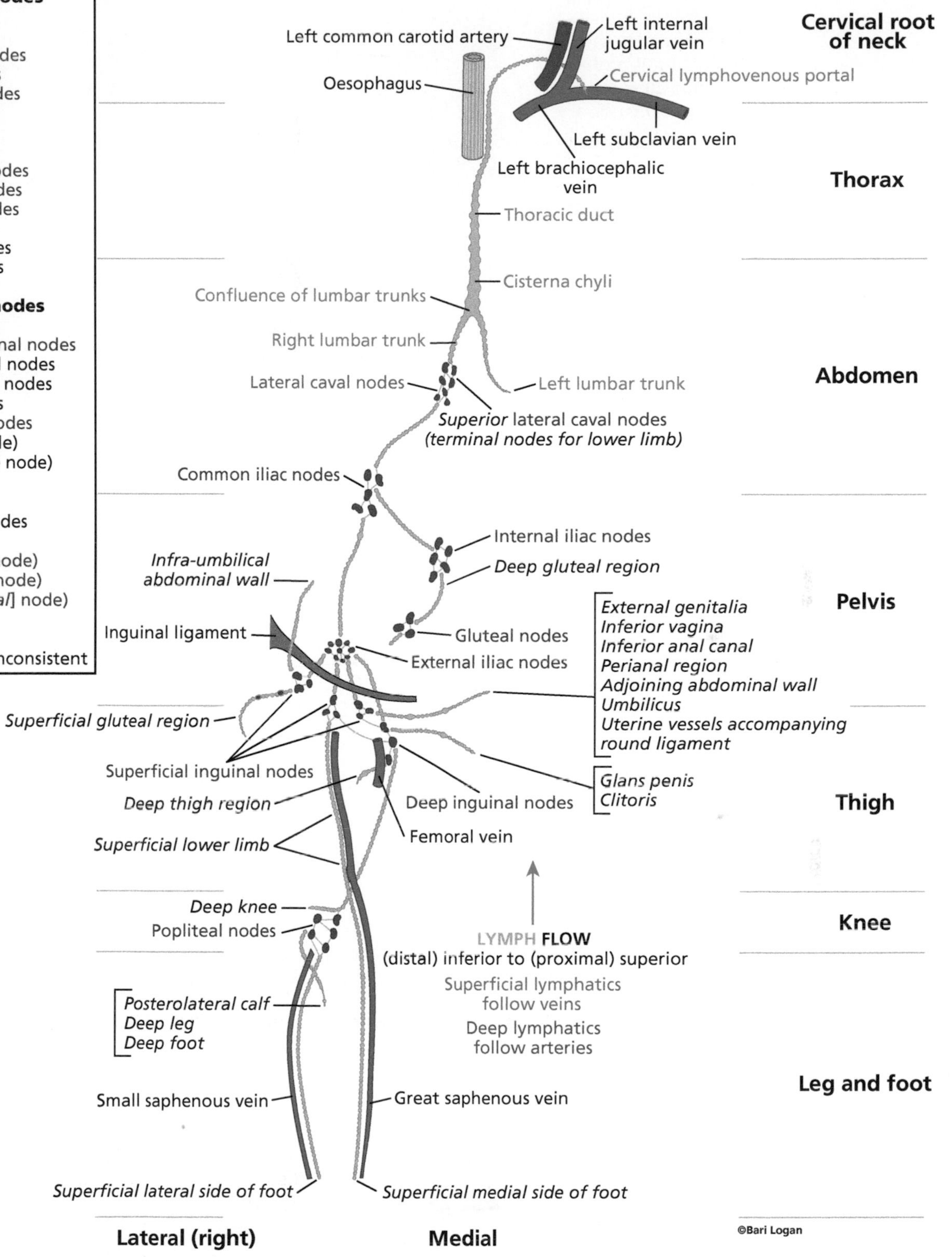

Left common carotid artery
Oesophagus
Left internal jugular vein
Cervical lymphovenous portal
Left subclavian vein
Left brachiocephalic vein
Thoracic duct
Cisterna chyli
Confluence of lumbar trunks
Right lumbar trunk
Left lumbar trunk
Lateral caval nodes
Superior lateral caval nodes (terminal nodes for lower limb)
Common iliac nodes
Internal iliac nodes
Deep gluteal region
Infra-umbilical abdominal wall
Gluteal nodes
External iliac nodes
Inguinal ligament
External genitalia
Inferior vagina
Inferior anal canal
Perianal region
Adjoining abdominal wall
Umbilicus
Uterine vessels accompanying round ligament
Superficial gluteal region
Superficial inguinal nodes
Deep thigh region
Deep inguinal nodes
Femoral vein
Glans penis
Clitoris
Superficial lower limb
Deep knee
Popliteal nodes
LYMPH FLOW (distal) inferior to (proximal) superior
Superficial lymphatics follow veins
Deep lymphatics follow arteries
Posterolateral calf
Deep leg
Deep foot
Small saphenous vein
Great saphenous vein
Superficial lateral side of foot
Superficial medial side of foot
Lateral (right)   Medial

Cervical root of neck
Thorax
Abdomen
Pelvis
Thigh
Knee
Leg and foot

©Bari Logan

Fig. 26 Schematic drawing (not to scale) of the lymphatic drainage of the right lower limb.

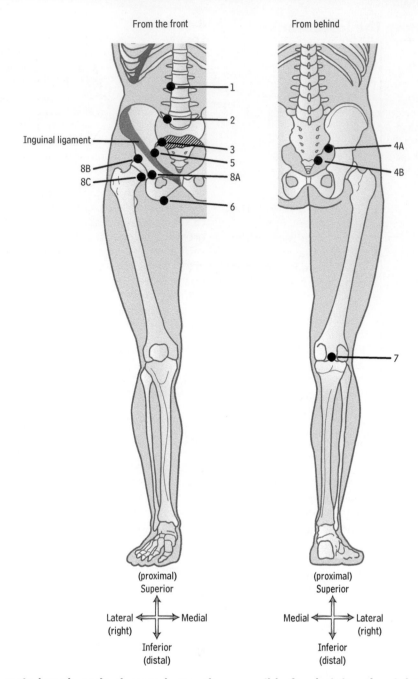

From the front

From behind

Inguinal ligament

1
2
3
5
8A
6
8B
8C

4A
4B
7

(proximal)
Superior

Lateral
(right)

Medial

Inferior
(distal)

(proximal)
Superior

Medial

Lateral
(right)

Inferior
(distal)

Fig. 27 Position of the main lymph node clusters (groups) responsible for draining the right lower limb.

1 Lateral caval nodes
Located **within the retroperitoneum** on the posterior abdominal wall, the **lateral caval nodes** occur on the **right side** of the body **flanking the vena cava**, hence (caval). Their counterparts, the **lateral aortic nodes,** occur on the **left side** of the body **flanking the aorta**, hence (aortic). Both groups of nodes, anterior to the medial margins of the psoas major muscles, diaphragmatic crura and sympathetic trunks, receive efferents from the common iliac nodes. There is moderate left-to-right crossover to nodes between the inferior vena cava and the aorta.

2 Common iliac nodes
Located **within the pelvis**, a cluster of normally **four to six nodes** scattered **around the common iliac artery**. Some nodes of this group occur inferior to the bifurcation of the aorta and anterior to the fifth lumbar vertebra or promontory of the sacrum. They receive efferents from the internal iliac nodes and external iliac nodes.

3 Internal iliac nodes
Located **deep within the pelvis** level with the lumbosacral intervertebral disc and anterior to the sacroiliac joint. These **nodes surround the internal iliac artery and vein** scattered between the commencement of the artery, at the common iliac bifurcation, and the superior margin of the greater sciatic notch. They receive efferents from the gluteal nodes.

4 Gluteal nodes
Located **deep within the pelvis** the gluteal nodes are **a subgroup of the internal iliac nodes** and **form two small clusters:**
4A. **Superior node**—normally a single node that occurs close to the intrapelvic part of the superior gluteal artery near to the border of the greater sciatic notch of the hip bone.
4B. **Inferior nodes**—normally two nodes that occur close to the inferior gluteal artery just inferior to the piriformis muscle. They drain the deep gluteal region.

5 External iliac nodes
Located **within the pelvis** posterior to the inguinal ligament midway between the anterior superior iliac spine of the hip bone and pubic symphysis. These nodes, normally **8–10 in number, form three clusters around the external iliac artery and vein** in a **lateral**, **medial** and **anterior*** position. They receive efferents from the superficial inguinal nodes and deep inguinal nodes.

6 Deep inguinal nodes
Located **deep in the anterior upper thigh** embedded **in the fat of the femoral triangle.** Normally **one to three nodes** in number, but may vary, lying **just medial to the femoral vein. Proximal node***—situated lateral in the femoral ring. **Intermediate node***—situated in the femoral canal. **Distal node**—situated just distal to the **saphenofemoral** junction. These nodes drain the glans penis, clitoris and deep thigh and receive efferents from the popliteal nodes and a few from the superficial inguinal nodes.

7 Popliteal nodes
Located **at the back of the knee** embedded **in the fat of the popliteal fossa.** Normally **six small nodes** laying **close to the popliteal vessels.** Some **superficial nodes** of the group occur near the termination of the small saphenous vein and some **deep nodes** lay between the popliteal artery and posterior aspect of the knee joint. This group of nodes drains the deep knee, posterolateral calf, deep leg and deep foot and receives efferents that accompany the small saphenous vein from the superficial lateral side of the leg and foot.

8 Superficial inguinal nodes
Located **superficially in the anterior upper thigh** embedded **in the subcutaneous fat of the femoral triangle**, these **nodes form three distinct cluster groups**. The **superomedial** and **superolateral** nodes, normally **five to six in number** situated just **distal and below the medial and lateral parts of the inguinal ligament**, and the **inferior nodes**, normally **four to five in number**, just **lateral to and along the termination of the great saphenous vein.**
8A. The **superomedial nodes** drain superficial lymphatics from the external genitalia, inferior vagina, inferior anal canal, perianal region, adjoining abdominal wall, umbilicus and the uterine vessels that accompany the round ligament.
8B. The **superolateral nodes** drain superficial lymphatics from the infraumbilical anterior abdominal wall and gluteal region.
8C. The **inferior nodes** receive efferents accompanying the great saphenous vein from the superficial lateral side of the leg and foot, except for the posterolateral calf.

Note: * denotes inconsistent structures.

Arteries

BRANCHES OF THE FEMORAL ARTERY

Giving off the following before becoming the popliteal
*   artery*
Superficial epigastric
Superficial circumflex iliac
Superficial external pudendal
Deep external pudendal
Profunda femoris, giving off
*   Lateral circumflex femoral*
*   Medial circumflex femoral*
*   Perforating*
Descending genicular

BRANCHES OF THE POPLITEAL ARTERY

Sural
Superior, middle and inferior genicular
Anterior tibial, giving off the following before becoming
*   the dorsalis pedis artery (see below)*
*   Posterior and anterior tibial recurrent*
*   Anterior medial and anterior lateral malleolar*
Posterior tibial, giving off
*   Circumflex fibularis*
*   Fibular (peroneal), giving off*
*   Nutrient to the fibula*
*   Perforating*
*   Communicating*
*   Lateral malleolar*
*   Calcanean*
*   Nutrient to the tibia*
*   Communicating*
*   Medial malleolar*
*   Calcanean*
*   Medial plantar (see below)*
*   Lateral plantar (see below)*

BRANCHES OF THE DORSALIS PEDIS ARTERY (Fig. 28)

Lateral dorsal
Medial dorsal
First dorsal metatarsal, giving off
*   Deep plantar (perforating) branch, to complete*
*   plantar arch*
*   Dorsal digital branch to medial side of great toe*
*   Dorsal digital branches of first cleft*

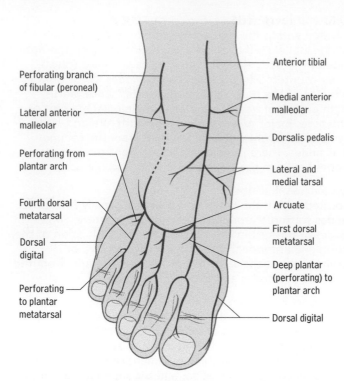

Fig. 28 Diagram of branches of the right dorsalis pedis artery, excluding muscular and most anastomotic branches; note that anastomoses from the perforating branch of the fibular (*peroneal*) artery may link up with the arcuate artery and enlarge to replace an absent dorsalis pedis artery.

Labels on figure:
Perforating branch of fibular (peroneal)
Lateral anterior malleolar
Perforating from plantar arch
Fourth dorsal metatarsal
Dorsal digital
Perforating to plantar metatarsal
Anterior tibial
Medial anterior malleolar
Dorsalis pedis
Lateral and medial tarsal
Arcuate
First dorsal metatarsal
Deep plantar (perforating) to plantar arch
Dorsal digital

Arcuate, giving off
*   Second dorsal metatarsal, giving off*
*   Perforating branches*
*   Dorsal digital branches to second cleft*
*   Third dorsal metatarsal, giving off*
*   Perforating branches*
*   Dorsal digital branches to third cleft*
*   Fourth dorsal metatarsal, giving off*
*   Perforating branches*
*   Dorsal digital branches to fourth cleft*
*   Dorsal digital branch to lateral side of fifth toe*

BRANCHES OF THE MEDIAL PLANTAR ARTERY

*Anastomotic branch to plantar digital artery of medial
   side of the great toe*
*Superficial digital branches to anastomose with first,
   second and third plantar metatarsal arteries*

BRANCHES OF THE LATERAL PLANTAR ARTERY (Fig. 29)

Plantar arch, giving off
   First plantar metatarsal, giving off
      Plantar digital artery to medial side of great toe
      Plantar digital arteries to first cleft
   *Second, third and fourth plantar metatarsal arteries,
      each giving off*
      *Plantar digital arteries to second, third and fourth
         clefts, respectively*
   Perforating branches
Plantar digital artery to lateral side of fifth toe

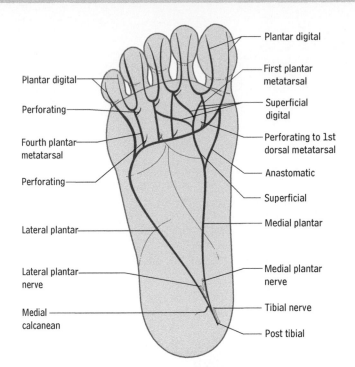

**Fig. 29 Diagram of branches of the right medial and
lateral plantar arteries (excluding muscular and most
anastomotic branches). The proximal parts of the
medial and lateral plantar nerves are shown in green
to indicate that the nerves lie on the internal sides of
their corresponding arteries.**

Index

Page numbers followed by "*f*" indicate figures.

Vessels
  afferent lymphatic, 165
  anterior tibial, 75, 75*f*, 104*f*
  circumflex femoral, 122, 122*f*
  femoral, 27*f*, 29, 29*f*–30*f*
  fibular *(peroneal)*, 104*f*
  lateral plantar, 101, 101*f*, 103*f*–104*f*, 106*f*–107*f*, 107, 110*f*
  lateral tarsal, 84*f*–85*f*, 85

  medial circumflex femoral, 21, 21*f*
  medial plantar, 100, 100*f*, 104*f*, 110*f*
  ovarian, 12*f*–13*f*, 13
  popliteal, 39, 39*f*
  posterior tibial, 75, 75*f*, 86*f*–87*f*, 104*f*
  profunda femoris, 21, 21*f*, 29, 29*f*–30*f*
  superficial circumflex iliac, 26, 26*f*

  superficial external pudendal, 26, 26*f*
  tibial, 40*f*–41*f*, 41
  see also Arteries; Veins

W
Weight bearing, 45, 89

Z
Zona orbicularis, 21, 21*f*, 123, 123*f*